60 IN 6: EVERYTHING YOUR MOTHER TOLD YOU TO DO

THE SHOCK JOCK OF WEIGHT LOSS BOOKS

DALE BONDANZA

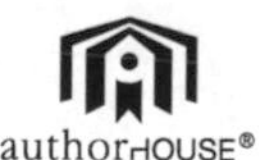

AuthorHouse™ LLC
1663 Liberty Drive
Bloomington, IN 47403
www.authorhouse.com
Phone: 1-800-839-8640

Published by AuthorHouse 06/26/2014

ISBN: 978-1-4969-1717-1 (sc)
ISBN: 978-1-4969-1716-4 (e)

Library of Congress Control Number: 2014910247

CONTENTS

FOREWORD

The foreword is where you're supposed to thank your inspiration for the work you're about to read. It's the last part of my book that I wrote. Normally, people thank their spouse, parents, family, or another cadre of people. After having thought about it for a few weeks I decided that if this is the first thing you're reading in my book than I may as well introduce you to me right up front. Who/What has helped me gain clarity, live healthy, and propelled me through more miles on the road than anything... Clearly, I'd like to thank my anger. Running has offset my anger management issues. Anger has helped me gut out more miles when my body said, "I think we're done now" than any other single factor in my life. Who am I most thankful to for having this grand life epiphany, losing the weight, getting and staying healthy? Easy answer. ME! That's who I'm thankful to. No one else has sweat, cried, and bled for me. I did these things. Others have helped. You'll read about them and they are angels with skin but in the end, who will turn your life around – YOU, no one else. No one else gives a crap. I made the choice! You have made your choices in the past and I hope after reading this book you will make new choices based on similar experiences to mine. Peace and Calm!

P.S. If you see me running Route 41 or Gulf Shore Blvd in Naples, FL please feel free to yell out something like, "keep running you fat bastard", "run faster fattie", "if you haven't hit 10 miles – keep going"... Don't be offended if I flip you off as a sign of love and respect because I would know you yelled because you read my book. If you see me running and grant me the ultimate honor of running with me even if it's only for a quarter of a mile or 5 miles I would love that too.

"I, Dale Bondanza, am not a licensed physician or health professional. This is a memoir of my personal experience with weight loss and not intended to serve as advice or guidance. Although, professionals were consulted, their advice and consultation was specific to me, and not generated for the use of the mass population. Before commencing any health regimen or weight loss journey, please contact your personal physician or health care professional." – Would you like to debate whether or not I actually wrote that sentence?

DISCLAIMER/APOLOGY! WHAT THIS BOOK IS/IS NOT! WHO IS THIS BOOK FOR?

I apologize for foul language, images, and truths that will offend you. I don't mean to shock as much as emphasize my points. I have decided to be blunt with this book, which may shock and or embarrass some of my family. While this is not my intention, it is unavoidable to tell my story – the full story of my journey. So, if you are a member of my family, you'll probably want to stop reading now (but thanks for buying a copy ☺). I value humor and I laugh at myself as much as at others; but make no mistake, this book is aimed at fatties of all kinds, sizes, shapes, and creeds. I will be insulting you, but I can empathize with you more than your personal trainer or doctor can. Why? 'Cause I've been there, been fat, had a problem, fixed it. So can you. Now quit your bitching and keep reading.

I need to cover an important theme of this book and it's based on my very limited knowledge of psychology. I understand I'm not a psychologist – not that I have anything against "shrinks." I think 80 percent of America needs to see a "shrink." It's important because it's the basis of my sarcasm, my attitude, and my success. Part of my undergraduate degree was a minor in Psychology and I've used quite a bit of it in my career. I've used the concepts of BF Skinner (famous psychologist from the early 20th century) related to reinforcement/punishment in many areas of my life, including my management of people who work for me as well as on myself to secure some of the changes I've made to get healthy and lose my weight. You must understand the difference between reinforcement and punishment.

You can have positive or negative of either, that is: positive reinforcement, negative reinforcement, positive punishment, or negative punishment. Negative means I'm taking something away and positive means I'm adding something. Let's use a couple examples. Positive punishment: when you touch a hot stove; you are positively punished because pain is added to your stimulus to remind you of the punishment for touching a hot stove. Negative punishment: the ultimate negative punishment is after yelling at your boss, and you find yourself being fired by Human Resources, thus removing your regular paycheck. Ouch! Let's talk reinforcement for a minute. Opposite of punishment, reinforcement is meant to incentivize a behavior (BF Skinner called this operant conditioning – Google it if you want to know more). So, you are removing something to reinforce a desired behavior. The desired behavior is to avoid getting in a fight with your significant other. The action taken was to clean up the mess in the kitchen before they get home. You've removed something (the mess) to reinforce the avoidance of an argument. Positive reinforcement is the addition of something to reinforce the behavior. Much easier concept...You exceed your sales quota and get a bonus at work. You got a bonus, thus reinforcing the behavior of exceeding your quota.

How am I going to motivate you to make this radical change in your lifestyle? I am going to use significant positive reinforcement. HOWEVER, coupled with this positive reinforcement, I'm going to use psychological concepts of positive punishment that may offend, shock, or anger you. GOOD! Use that shock or anger to motivate you to cease the behavior that's making you fat and unhealthy. As stated earlier, the goal of punishment is to decrease the behavior that precedes the punishment. The behavior is eating poorly, not exercising, and not focusing on an overall healthy lifestyle. You will be mentally and verbally punished by the addition of my harsh words. I will, however, reinforce positively, your behaviors that lead you away from fatness and into healthiness.

This book is my account of my inspiration and my journey. This book is about how I lost 60 pounds in 6 months doing exactly what our mother's told us to do when we were kids. (FYI: It was actually 85 pounds in about 9.5 months but 60 in 6 made a better book title.) This is not a "how to guide" for losing weight. It is my story and what inspired me, pained me, and eventually motivated me. This book is a vehicle for me to continue my healing and keep my head screwed on straight. Over the course of six months and beyond I saw how my journey affected people and the closer I got to my goals the more I felt I needed to share my story. Ergo, *60 in 6: Everything Your Mother Told You To Do.* This book is my first full book, but I sincerely hope it's not my last. When I was coming up with a title for the book, I had to admit to myself and to my mother, that my tag line for the book was certainly not everything my mother told us (me or my four brothers) to do growing up; but it is what most mothers tell their children. Growing up in Buffalo, New York in a middle income, 75 percent Italian household, it was considered insulting to not finish any food that was put in front of you. "There are starving children in Africa." I have come to believe that my story is inspirational. This book is intended to inspire you to lose weight and get healthy. It's within your control, no one else's! It's not a "how to guide." It's not medically researched or clinically based (although I'll give references when I use them). It's not a magic bullet. There is no such thing. Trust me, I've looked and researched and tried them all. This book will not change your life overnight but it will change your opinion if you keep an open mind. You're NOT alone. There are millions of people including me on your side. Together, we can make America thinner and healthier and return it to the status as the sex symbol of the world instead of just the wealth, wasteful, and gluttony status we maintain today.

If you're reading this then there's an 80 percent chance you are fat. If you're not fat (to be defined in a minute), you probably were at some point or may be in future; therefore, this book is you. I guarantee you 100 percent that you know someone who is fat. So, if you can say, "I know this guy who lost all this weight and I believe you can to," then please bring my inspiration to others and your good karma will be rewarded. If you're a skinny marathoner or someone from Kenya, you don't need my help getting skinny. If you're in your 20s, you probably won't listen to me anyway because you still have a fast metabolism and think you have all the answers anyway. If you are more than 30 years old, then you will be able to relate to and appreciate the last six months of my life. If you are the parents of someone less than 30 years old, who is a fatty, you may also be able to help them without them even knowing it. Basically, if you care about anyone who is fat, including yourself, and you want to change it, then keep reading. Here is the Body Mass Index (BMI) chart. I can already hear the complaining beginning. Yes, the chart is the same for both men and women. So, if you're an average man (5'10" = 70 inches tall) then ideally your range can be anywhere from 132 pounds to 174 pounds. Realistically, the healthy, left most columns are broken into seven columns/indexes. It's not unfair to say, while it may be sexist, that most men will fit into the top 3 1/2 columns or a BMI index of 22.5 to 25. Most women should be in a BMI index from 19 up to 22.5. What I can most certainly tell you is that at my current weight (155 pounds at 5'10") with 13 percent body fat, I'm healthy, athletic, and satisfied with my appearance for the first time in over 40 years.

In general, if you are one pound over the max then you are fat. Greater than 10 percent = "overweight," greater than 20 percent = "obese," greater than 30 percent = "morbid obesity." This is a general rule – not as scientific as the chart above. We'll address excuses in the next chapter, as I'm sure yours are similar to the ones I've had my whole life. This book is primarily targeted at people who are in the obese and morbidly obese categories.

BMI Chart	19	20	21	22	23	24	25	26	27	28	29	30	31	32	33	34	35	36	37	38	39	40	41	42	43	44	45	46	47	48	49	50	51	52	53	54
Height																																				
Inches	Body Weight (Pounds)																																			
58	91	96	100	105	110	115	119	124	129	134	138	143	148	153	158	162	167	172	177	181	186	191	196	201	205	210	215	220	224	229	234	239	244	248	253	258
59	94	99	104	109	114	119	124	128	133	138	143	148	153	158	163	168	173	178	183	188	193	198	203	208	212	217	222	227	232	237	242	247	252	257	262	267
60	97	102	107	112	118	123	128	133	138	143	148	153	158	163	168	174	179	184	189	194	199	204	209	215	220	225	230	235	240	245	250	255	261	266	271	276
61	100	106	111	116	122	127	132	137	143	148	153	158	164	169	174	180	185	190	195	201	206	211	217	222	227	232	238	243	248	254	259	264	269	275	280	285
62	104	109	115	120	126	131	136	142	147	153	158	164	169	175	180	186	191	196	202	207	213	218	224	229	235	240	246	251	256	262	267	273	278	284	289	295
63	107	113	118	124	130	135	141	146	152	158	162	169	175	180	186	191	197	203	208	214	220	225	231	237	242	248	254	259	265	270	278	282	287	293	299	304
64	110	116	122	128	134	140	145	151	157	163	169	174	180	186	192	197	204	209	215	221	227	232	238	244	250	256	262	267	273	279	285	291	296	302	308	314
65	114	120	126	132	138	144	150	156	162	168	174	180	186	192	198	204	210	216	222	228	234	240	246	252	258	264	270	276	282	288	294	300	306	312	3118	324
66	118	124	130	136	142	148	155	161	167	173	179	186	192	198	204	210	216	223	229	235	241	247	253	260	266	272	278	284	291	297	303	309	315	322	328	334
67	121	127	134	140	146	153	159	166	172	178	185	191	198	204	211	217	223	230	236	242	249	255	261	268	274	280	287	293	299	306	312	319	325	331	338	344
68	125	131	138	144	151	158	164	171	177	184	190	197	203	210	216	223	230	236	243	249	256	262	269	276	282	289	295	302	308	315	322	328	335	341	348	354
69	128	135	142	149	155	162	169	176	182	189	196	203	209	216	223	230	236	243	250	257	263	270	277	284	291	297	304	311	318	324	331	338	345	351	358	365
70	132	139	146	153	160	167	174	181	188	195	202	209	216	222	229	236	243	250	257	264	271	278	285	292	299	306	313	320	327	334	341	348	355	362	369	376
71	136	143	150	157	165	172	179	186	193	200	208	215	222	229	236	243	250	257	265	272	279	286	293	301	308	315	322	329	338	343	351	358	365	372	379	386
72	140	147	154	162	169	177	184	191	199	206	213	221	228	235	242	250	258	265	272	279	287	294	302	309	316	324	331	338	346	353	361	368	375	383	390	397
73	144	151	159	166	174	182	189	197	204	212	219	227	235	242	250	257	265	272	280	288	295	302	310	318	325	333	340	348	355	363	371	378	386	393	401	408
74	148	155	163	171	179	186	194	202	210	218	225	233	241	249	256	264	272	280	287	295	303	311	319	326	334	342	350	358	365	373	381	389	396	404	412	420
75	152	160	168	176	184	192	200	208	216	224	232	240	248	256	264	272	279	287	295	303	311	319	327	335	343	351	359	367	375	383	391	399	407	415	423	431
76	156	164	172	180	189	197	205	213	221	230	238	246	254	263	271	279	287	295	304	312	320	328	336	344	353	361	369	377	385	394	402	410	418	426	435	443

Legend
Healthy
Overweight
Obese
Morbid Obese

Let's discuss, for a few minutes, your fatness. If, based on the charts and discussion above you're fat, than let's discuss some basic truths... FAT = UGLY. FAT = LAZY. You may not be an ugly person, but your fat is. You can be "not fat" and lazy but if you are fat you are most certainly lazy. You are not "pleasantly plump," portly, heavy, "a few extra pounds," bigger boned, or husky. There is not more of you to love. You are disgusting to yourself and others. You know it, they know it, and so does everyone else. I'm not saying they don't love you (especially if they are your family), but fat is not the new skinny. Think of something disgusting to you. Maybe it's pornography, maybe a serial rapist, maybe 9/11, maybe liberals, conservatives, terrorists, lawyers, etc., being fat should disgust you more than whatever you chose above; but it probably doesn't because you, like me, have/had an addiction to being fat. It's called "comfort food" for a reason. It contains high amounts of fats and carbohydrates. It contains an unending amount of sodium and more chemical additives than you care to know about. But damn it, does it taste good! Driving by at McDonald's for a fatty is like an addict driving by a sign that says "free crack." Does this addiction need a 12-step program? It just might. I'll help you identify that in a few minutes. Since we're still discussing your fatness, I want to make a couple additional points about this book and my story. I said earlier that this book is not a "how to guide" on weight loss because, in general, I believe all diets are bullshit. If you only have to lose five pounds or, oh my God, 10 pounds, I'm not sure why you're reading this book. There is a "diet" out there for you somewhere. However, diets are still bullshit because the basic formula has not changed since the days of the caveman. "More calories out than in" is the only formula you'll ever need to remember. I, nor you, will care about proteins, carbohydrates, sodium, sugars, chemicals, etc. to get you skinny; we are going to focus on the basics. We are going to talk about your caloric intake. We are going to talk about making a life- changing decision to be healthy, to lose weight, and to conquer your addiction to fatness.

EXCUSES

I'm certain that I could write a book with nothing but excuses. For more than 20 years I offered every excuse possible. This portion of my book will be a stream of consciousness. The most important sentence in this chapter is an old familiar phrase. "Excuses are like assholes! Everyone's got one and they all stink!" There are many people who we joke about and say, "Oh he thinks his shit doesn't stink." Basic human anatomy; all shit stinks, all excuses are a parallel. Get it? Good! Move on.

The basic reason I love this chapter is because I wrote the first chapter in about two sittings. I then closed Microsoft Word for about six months, not to open it again to this manuscript because I continued to make excuses about even finishing this healing text. Why? Why would I not want to share my experience? Was I afraid others would look negatively at me? Was I afraid others would be able to beat me in a race? Was I really worried about how the book "ends" which is what I told most people for the last six months? "I'm not sure how the book should end. I'm not sure if it should end with me doing a marathon, with me returning to Key West, with the surgery that I know I need…" Just like losing the fat, I procrastinated because I wanted the perfect answer. SHOCKER!!! There isn't one. It took me 40-plus years to have the epiphany to get healthy. Why would I think explaining it would take any less?

I will try and rattle off all of the excuses I've used, heard, or experienced during my journey. I can say, with no uncertainty that they are all bullshit! There is no excuse for your fatness. There's not a medical, psychological, physiological, social, emotional, or faith-based reason that you can't solve or ask someone to help you solve. You just don't have the faith in yourself to climb the hill. It's in you! The tears of joy you get when you get to the top of that hill is like no other feeling. To know you kicked ass, took life by the balls and said, "NO," I control you, not the other way around is profound and self inspirational. OK, here goes (again, trying stream of consciousness)…

I was born this way. It's because of my cultural heritage (pick one… Puerto Rican, Swedish, Black, Latino, Nordic, Italian…). I have a thyroid problem. I'm depressed. I'm on medication. I have psychological issues to losing weight. I have bigger bones. I workout, so I have a lot of muscle mass that makes my BMI higher than it really is. The kids have to take priority and I don't have time. I don't have time! I work 12–18 hours a day. I have a long commute to work. I'm not built to run. I could never do what you did to get skinny/healthy. I'm not that disciplined. I like myself the way I am. I think I look pretty good with the weight. I'm still in very good cardio shape, despite my fat. My husband/wife says I'm not fat. I'm not as fat as others (my friends, family, etc…). I don't have time to workout. I don't have time to eat healthy. I can't run, my knees are bad. It's too expensive to eat healthy. Our society doesn't promote healthy living. I really like cheesecake. I can't run. My hips are bad. I don't have time. I need my sleep. I really love beer. I can't run, my ankles are bad. I really love chocolate. I can't run. My shoulders hurt when I run. I really just don't have an extra hour in my day. I'm allergic to sweat (no really, I am). Why should I get healthy, I'm not going to live forever anyway. What's the point? I don't have the time. I enjoy my life and the way I'm living it – why should I change? I can't afford a gym membership. I have low self-esteem. I pay for a gym membership, but I don't like the people there; they are intimidating, they are all muscle heads, they use it as a social club, they… they… they… ("Man this is getting annoying! Is anyone else as pissed off yet as I am writing this?)

You know you've used many of these; and I've used almost all of them except the kid's lines because as I write this book, at the age of 44, I have never had any children (my choice – not another excuse). HOWEVER, that still allows me to comment on your excuse because the same basic formulas still apply.

Your excuses are bullshit! You CAN make the time! It's not expensive to live and eat properly (although if you have money, you absolutely have no excuses whatsoever)! You don't have to belong to a gym (although it helps). You don't have to pay for a dietician (although it'd help). You don't have to have a personal trainer (although it helps). You CAN make the time! You think it will take away from your other activities? BULLSHIT! It will enhance them, significantly. It will give you more time back to be better at everything else you do from work to family to relationships. It is an investment; in yourself, that pays dividends/rewards like no other program you've ever seen. Like all investments, it does require you to give up something to get something larger in return, but the inside secret is no matter how much you invest, the return (unlike the stock market and economy) will ALWAYS pay positive dividends. You will feel better, look better, and be a better person. Sounds almost unrealistic, sounds improbable, sounds like bullshit! It's not! Proper diet and exercise will change your life... Sounds like something your mother would say, doesn't it? It is and it's that simple.

Let me try and address some of the excuses you used above. There are probably a ton of additional excuses I didn't list, but I still think the answers to most of them will be the same. And, throughout the book I will address many of these issues, even if I don't address them here. Or, more likely, I will touch on them here and go into more detail later. You may have even seen a theme in the "excuses" above. That is, time is our enemy. It is the ally of laziness. It is the enemy of exercise. Not really, but that's how people make them out. Time is not the enemy, but it is a variable that you must control. What makes time easier for me to control than other people? Maybe it's because I'm fairly OCD (obsessive compulsive disorder). Maybe it's because I'm fairly anal about everything I do (a Freudian psychology reference – for those who think it means something different). Time is not the enemy! FAT is the ENEMY! Don't confuse the two. A popular religious phrase is "idleness is a tool of the devil." This can work in reverse as well. That is, you think you're so busy that nothing else can possibly interrupt your precious schedule. Again, this is the FAT talking. If you're a man, it's the estrogen in your system talking. If you're a woman, it's the estrogen in your system talking. Don't let the FAT or the hormones take control. You have control, not the fat, not the hormones. You're going to tell me you don't sleep enough as it is, I can't take any more time away from my sleep. Guess what? BULLSHIT! Get used to it. You're going to hear the same answer time and time again in this book. STOP MAKING FUCKING EXCUSES AND JUST DO IT! I hate to quote Nike and they'll probably sue me for it, but it really is a phrase that applies to you losing the weight. You can do it, you will do it, and you must do it.

You need a minimum of an extra 30 minutes in every day of the week (that's 3.5 hours / week). This is the minimum and I tell you with God as my witness you can find 3.5 hours within your 168 hour week. That's two percent of your total week. Quick aside if I didn't already mention it. I will help you do a LOT of math in this book. Numbers do not lie. (Mark Twain popularized, "Lies, damned lies, and statistics.") They are facts, they are not subjective. They are what they are. They are irrefutable. You need to know numbers to understand your battle with fat. You DO NOT need to be a math genius. I know many people just took a huge sigh of relief. No, math is not something you need to be good at, but you do need to understand numbers. I said 30 minutes every day was the minimum, I guess I put off the obvious long enough. Exactly, how fat are you? Your fatness is directly proportional to the amount of time and energy you need to invest to rid yourself of it. From the title of the book, 60 in 6, I will tell you, in all honesty, I had to find about 12 to 14 hours in my weekly schedule to conquer my fat-bastard self. Holy shit you're saying. Where am I going to find two hours EVERY day (eight percent) of my week to get healthy? I know it sounds like a lot, but once you get there you'll be so happy; you'll actually be mad you were wasting the time on whatever activity you're about to put behind you. It's not from one place, it's from many places. You'll find it. Relax!! I'll tell you how I did it; and while you'll resist my explanations, you'll accept it after you calm down a little and take a breath. You may even stop reading this chapter for a few days until you pick it back up because you're going to be mad at me for calling you out on your bullshit excuses. You're not kidding anyone except yourself; so, unless you're reading this out loud you're not bullshitting anyone except yourself, so stop it!

Sleep – don't need as much as you think. "But science says I need six hours, seven hours, eight hours…" Sure, I'll buy that and I promise you'll get it… eventually. Once you give up some sleep (in the beginning) to get healthy, eventually you'll actually be able to get more sleep, get more restful sleep, deeper sleep and it will (as I already said) pay dividends you didn't expect. Give up a little sleep now for more sleep later. It's true, it works.

And the No. 1 killer of Americans time… here it comes, don't get pissy, finish the paragraph before you throw the book against the wall… TV, the boob tube (as your mother called it), the box, cable, Comcast, Dish, Hulu, video games, anything that causes you to sit on the couch, the lazy chair, the love seat, the floor, etc… in front a screen that you say allows you to "de-stress" from your day and vegetate just to relieve your brain of its stress from the day. Your largest amount of weekly time will most likely come from this incredibly wasteful activity. It did for me. When you actually document, as you will, how much time you spend watching TV or "having it on in the background" or listening to it on sleep timer as you're going to bed, you will shock yourself. It's ALL WASTED TIME you could be losing weight, you fat pig!

Here's another one that's going to tick off some folks… Hanging out, going out with friends, or the easiest excuse, "the kids." I can't steal two hours per week from my kids (or my friends or my spouse or my significant other). OK, sit down; this is where it gets brutal again. "Kids" as a word will be used as the generic reference for all the groups I previously stated. Do you know what's worse than stealing two hours per week from your kids for the next eight months (70 hours if you're counting)? You being DEAD earlier than you should be from obesity, diabetes, heart failure, or other co-morbid conditions associated with obesity. You are a HORRIBLE, SHITTY role model for your kids if you are fat. They will think it's OK to be a fat, out-of-shape loser; and while EVERYONE wants their kids to have it better than they did, you are sending the opposite message when you can't control your own life. You want to steal about seven years away from your own life (away from your kids' life) – that's what "science" will tell you you're giving up on average. That's 61,320 hours given up for your fatness. So 70 hours over the next eight months seems like a solid investment to save the 61,320 hours you'll get on the back end. Again, it's simple math. Here's another fun one.

I don't know who's going to be more pissed at this paragraph, the employers or the people who are so loyal to their employers…Yep, you guessed it. You can sacrifice two hours a week from your job. OK, this is going to be challenging to explain to 60 percent of the audience reading this book. Let me address the 40 percent first. I believe that 40 percent of the people reading my book are salaried / exempt employees who are paid the same amount (weekly, monthly, annually), whether they work 37.5 hours per week or 80 hours per week. While I'm being kind, I think we can all acknowledge that even if you're only slated to work 37.5 hours per week (a 40-hour week with 30 minutes of lunch break per day,) you probably put in more than 37.5 hours. If you're the "typical salaried American" working a 40-hour week, you probably put it between 50–60 hours (on average). This is time spent "in the office" but I can guarantee you as a people and project manager for the last 20 years that while you're "in the office", that 50–60 hours is not spent 100 percent of the time "working," "counting beans," "punching numbers," "being creative," "making or saving your company money." There's two hours in there of time spent bullshitting about your kids, the football game, politics, or a multitude of other subjects. You can find two hours EASILY!

If they want to chat, tell them to join you at the gym or on the local high school track. You'll be respected as a leader and as someone who's taking control of their life. You will be an inspiration to your colleagues. Now, let me address the other 60 percent. These are people who make an hourly (non-exempt) wage. You are a waitress/waiter making $2.50/ hour + tips. You're a construction worker, EMT, fire-fighter making $12/ hour for your 40 hours of work, and if you get caught bullshitting or not "truly working" for that 40 hours, some asshole supervisor "docks your pay." How do you find two hours per week when you're paid for every second you work? Similar to what I said about the "salaried" employees above. When you are not "on the clock" you "stick around" your job after you've officially punched out or before you clock in. Even if it's for 12 minutes before and 12 minutes after your shift (that's 24 minutes per day or 120 minutes over five days ergo two hours).

You stick around for a cigarette, a drink, to chat about the pain in the butt customer, or the jerk boss, or the dumb patient, citizen, etc...It's 24 minutes a day (24 MINUTES) of <u>your life</u> you're taking back, taking control to make your life better. And remember, you're only taking it back for the next eight months (give or take). Once you've figured it out, you'll be even more productive during your shift than you are today because you'll be healthier, more fit, stronger, and smarter than you are today thus benefiting you AND your employer. OK, go ahead, throw the book at the wall and tell me I'm full of shit I don't know your job, your boss, your co-workers (hell maybe you are the boss and you're saying, "I hope my employees aren't reading this")… Once you calm down, take a breath, and bring your blood pressure back under control you will think about 24 minutes a day. Hell, you just spent almost that much time throwing this book at the wall, going to the fridge to grab a drink or a piece of food before coming back to finish the paragraph. PUT THE CANDY BAR DOWN FATTY! When you get ticked at me next time, try some breathing exercises… Remember Lamas class you took when you were having kids? Remember Yoga class breathing? Pant like a dog, whatever helps fill those lungs with oxygen and lower that blood pressure.

<u>Where my 14 hours / week came from (in general):</u>
Sleep – 4 hours / week
TV – six hours / week
Hanging Out / Going Out with friends (the kids if that applies) - two hours / week
Work – two hours / week

OK, let's hit a few others in quick succession… I beat you up pretty well in the last few pages, I'll make the next few hurt a little less, I hope… Cultural heritage… Find me a race (ethnic) of purely fat humans (besides Americans). Is more than 50 percent of the group fat? Guess what, yes, there's plenty! As Americans, we should not be proud to be in this top 10 list with countries like Nauru, Micronesia, Tonga, Kuwait, Samoa, Niue, Palau… Do you even know where all these countries are? I had to admit I had to look up Niue. Looks like a fun place for a visit! (Raised eyebrow, emocon!). Once you Google map this island, you will see some of the other obese cultures that surround it… Niue is up to two flights a week into their country – I'm serious about that – that's per their own website. You, as an American, should be disgusted to be on this list. Are you? When I first started getting crap from my doctor about my weight I said, "Doc, that's why I see a short fat Italian doctor (just like me – Italian mostly). You wanna be the pot or the kettle, Doc?" Cultural heritage has almost nothing to do with your weight issues. Lessons you learned about as a kid from your Jamaican, Puerto Rican, Jewish, Italian, German, Irish parent may have influenced your youth and helped push you into fatness, but you're a big boy or girl now (literally and figuratively). Grow up!

I have a psychological problem… OK, I said in the beginning, I'm not a doctor and I only pretended to be one when I was drunk in a bar somewhere. You may truly have psych issues. You may be depressed, schizophrenic, bi-polar, general anxiety disorder, schizoaffective, PTSD, panic attacks, phobias, OCD, ADHD, personality disorders, mood disorders, or others. You will blame "the meds" for making you fat and in some cases the chemistry is true and "the meds" can make you fat, weak, tired, lethargic, more down than you were before "the meds." In general, "the meds" or your therapy is designed to try and return you to a "normal life." Part of this return to "normal life" is giving you the energy to do something, anything more than you're doing today is considered exercise because it's something more than you're doing normally. Hey, I didn't say this was going to be easy. I will say repeatedly, there is no magic formula. If there was, someone would have found it and be a billionaire by now. You can overcome your mental illness, even if you need help. You can walk to the corner. You can eventually walk to the next corner, in a couple of weeks you may walk fast or even in-line or roller skate to the corner. Again, if you walk down your stairs one more time per day than you do now, then you're doing more exercise than you're doing now. Keep it up, you're doing great!

I have a medical issue, thyroid problem, glandular issue, cancer, heart disease, COPD, I'm disabled… I mentioned the lack of MD after my name right? Same as above, they have meds to help you return to as normal a life as possible. Cancer – let's talk to Lance Armstrong (ignore the whole doping thing – get on a bike with one nut and ride around the block fatty). I'm sure a lawyer at some point will advise me to include the standard "gym membership phrase" about consulting your doctor before beginning any exercise program to make sure you're capable of doing it without killing yourself. Fair enough, do that so you don't sue my ass. After you've done that, do as I said in the last paragraph and simply walk to the corner for me. Do it every day this week, one time per day. Next week, do the same thing (maybe even with a little spring in your step). Repeat.

I like myself the way I am. *NO, you don't, remember you're reading this to yourself; so stop lying.* My wife/husband/partner doesn't think I'm fat. *Yes they do, but because they love you and have their own insecurities, they won't admit it to you.* Check the chart from the previous chapter. You know if you're fat. I'm not as fat as other people I know. "As fat" is the key word there. My knees, ankles, hips, etc… are bad – I can't walk, run, elliptical, bike, etc… I get shin splits, cramps, diarrhea, aches, and pains. You need a personal trainer, a coach, a dietician…These are all lousy excuses. Go volunteer at a few 5K races. When you see the 60, 70, 80-plus year-old men and women running in these races, you should take that excuse and shove it where the sun doesn't shine. Anyone can elliptical. It is the lowest form of impact on the joints and while I will discuss running ad nausea in this book all cardio applies. I have bigger bones. *That would be true if all your bones were in your ass.* They're not, go exercise. Gym memberships – I can't afford them – *that's fine because you don't need one.* It helps, but it's not completely necessary. Gym memberships – I have one but I don't like the people there. Don't worry, they don't like you either. Your fat inspires them to keep working harder but your fat disgusts them. You feel intimidated by them for one reason or another… Guess what, as you lose weight, gain speed, or healthiness, and gain self-confidence, suddenly you'll start to understand "the other side." One of my favorites… I'm in great cardio shape despite my weight problem. I have seen a number of people in spinning classes (including the actual instructors) that are overweight but can out-spin me and other true athletes like we're still morbidly obese. This does not outweigh their weight problem... Some will say, there's proof you can be in good cardio shape and still be fat. Yes, you can be in great cardio shape and have a 5,000 calorie a day diet because you love chocolate, alcohol, fried foods, cheese, carbs, etc... You're using one aspect of your like to justify another. You're enabling your own disillusion with your problem. If you have a great heart rate and blood pressure, but a gut that makes you look pregnant (whether you're a man or a woman) you need to address your issue. Your body is in turmoil if this case applies to you. You must be nicer to your body. It'll thank you later. It's funny to say, "The body is evil; it must be punished," but the reality is that you've punished it enough. It's time to love it a little.

I have another favorite that I honestly have a tougher time answering, but listen to my answer and then modify it based on your perspective. I'm not compiling the Bible on weight loss but I am sharing what I know works and what can help you help yourself. "I don't have time to eat healthy... It's too expensive to eat healthy... It's easy and cheap to eat off the dollar menu at McDonald's." The reason this is a tough one to answer for me is because this was one of my addictions. McDonald's and I were asshole buddies for a number of my drunken years. I had more Mickey D meals at 2 a.m., (after the bars closed) than I had during normal hours for many years. As you may know (if you're a current or former drinker) nothing goes better with mass quantities of alcohol than fats, carbs, and grease. YUM! "I don't have time," is bullshit because it takes no less time to eat healthy than it does to eat poorly.

You can say McDonald's is quick and making a chicken breast with rice takes 45 minutes, but I will also show you in later chapters how I condensed this process into a few hours per week and thus ended up saving more time in the end. Cheap versus expensive to be healthy... I'm not going to deny that when I had my original epiphany I was in the field of IT (Information Technology) and I was gainfully employed as a consultant. So, while there is some truth to the statement that "the only thing money can't buy is poverty," the opposite of "money can't buy happiness," is true as well. It doesn't buy happiness, but it can sure enable it. Fresh Market and Whole Foods and Trader Joe's are stores that healthy people die to be near. And, it's with good reason. Unfortunately, the prices at these stores are insane and while I'm a firm believer in "you get what you pay for," that doesn't help the person reading this book saying, "Great, I was all excited to lose the weight and now you're going to tell me I can't afford it." Not true. Let me not give away future chapters, but let's focus on the key words "portion control." Do you know how much a "serving" of ANYTHING is? After reading this book you will NEVER pick up another item of food at the supermarket and not read the two most important things on the label (serving size and calories per serving). If you do those things going forward, you will lose weight; and you don't have to change your food unless you have the desire/ability to. Again, the course I will describe to you, that I took, involved a fairly radical makeover of my life, diet, and plan, but you can vary this depending on your needs.

Wrap up excuses… "I'm not disciplined," "I'm not built to run," "I have a long commute to work," "What's the point." Disciplined… HA, me either, why do you think I was a FAT BASTARD for 41 years. I was lazy and didn't care until I hit rock bottom, not dissimilar from a junkie/alcoholic. I will teach you to be disciplined and it will take some time, but you will learn and you will be able to walk away from this book with practical guides to help you. I'm not built to run? Are you a human being (homosapien)? Then guess what, you were "Born to Run." You were born with a natural instinct to run. AFTER you get done with this book please pick up a copy of "Born To Run" by Christopher McDougall about the tribe of super athletes and the greatest race the world has ever seen. I was skeptical when I first was introduced to the book by a friend, but after finishing it I was a changed man on my perspective of running. What's the point? If you haven't figured out the point I implore you to put the book down now and get naked and stand in front of a full-length mirror for the next 20 minutes and come back and pick up this book. If you still don't get the point than either you're right and you can put the book on the shelf, never to be read again, or you need to repeat the process until you realize that you really are a fat, disgusting, pig. I have a long commute to work… Really? See my previous section about saving 24 minutes per day (minimum). You can find 24 minutes every day of the week. If you can't find 24 minutes, go stand in front of the mirror again.

Another favorite I hear from bodybuilders or those muscle heads at the gym… The BMI chart doesn't apply to me because of the amount of muscle mass I have. They're correct, the BMI chart does not take muscle mass of a body builder into consideration. IF, that's a HUGE IF, a bodybuilder is ripped with muscle but still is fat, than all I can say is cut out the steroids and do some planks and you'll be back into fighting shape soon enough. One pound of rocks is the same weight as one pound of feathers. Unlike you, however, the feathers are not as "dense" as the rocks.

Here's a little more math for my muscle head friend above. Muscle boy probably won't understand this but have your kindergarten teacher explain it to you. Body fat is an important concept in weight loss. You must measure it at the beginning of your journey so you know where you are. The reason I don't focus much on it is because I'm advocating an overall healthy lifestyle, and the method of losing the bulk of the weight comes from cardio AND weightlifting. You cannot lose a massive amount of weight without adding some muscle. You would look like a deflated truck tire and not achieve the benefits of a god/goddess like body that I've been telling you about.

The density of mammalian skeletal muscle is 1.06 g/ml.

The density of adipose tissue (fat) is about 0.9 g/ml

Therefore, muscle is about (1.06/0.92=) 1.15 times more dense than fat. So you're looking at about a 15 percent difference between the same weight of muscle and fat. So, let's take an easy example and say you're 400 pounds of fat (damn, you are a disgusting beast) and you're simply trying to get down to 200 (this is a 6-foot tall male by the way). And 200 pounds is still too big (I'd have him shoot for 180 pounds)' but we'll give him credit for cutting his weight in half and we'll tackle the last 20 pounds later. So 15 percent of 400 pounds equals 60 pounds. This is oversimplified for purposes of the book because nothing is absolute. If this whale went from 400 pounds down to 200 pounds exclusively through cardio and did zero weightlifting, he would look like a Shar-pei dog. Naturally, he will follow my advice and do weight lifting while doing the cardio. Will he add 60 pounds of muscle? Doubtfully. Will he add half of that amount? Hopefully! Therefore, at 200 pounds this former whale is now a hunk because he has an extra 30 pounds of muscle that makes him look as defined as Sly Stallone in Rocky. Part of the challenge I speak about in this book is that depending on the age when you start your journey, you will still have some similarities to our Shar-pei friend pictured below; however, loose skin can be dealt with. Your skin will retract (some) over time. The muscle you're gaining will help fill it out.

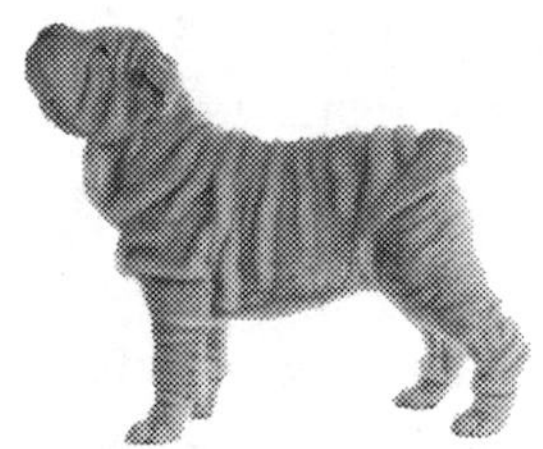

As you can imagine, while I was writing this book and talking to folks about its style of negative reinforcement and positive affirmations, I was confronted with even more excuses. While I'll continue to write, I reserve the right to come back and add "good excuses" as I progress. For instance, "Dale, don't you believe that you can be overweight and still fit." It's worth noting, this was said to me while I was running with the person. So, my kneejerk was to insultingly yell at the person, NO but I bit my tongue, pretended like I didn't hear the question and kept running, but thought about it over the next mile or so. I concluded, thinking back over my weight-loss journey, that I encountered plenty of people that fell into this category.

The No. 1 and No. 2 examples that I can remember are from the gym where I lost the majority of my weight (Hillsborough Racquet and Fitness Club in Hillsborough, NJ). The No. 1 example was a guy there who taught spin. He was probably late 40s or early 50s and he led a spin class at least once a week. He was probably about 6 feet, 1 inch tall and probably about 250+/- pounds. He was "in shape" because as I've defined above "round" IS a shape. He had a beer belly larger than anything I've ever had, even in my best drinking days. While I'm in better shape now than I was then, I still could not have kept up with his spinning class at his pace. Therefore, my conclusion is, "Yes, you can be **cardio fit** and overweight." HOWEVER, with the huge belly while he may be "fit" he is not "healthy." Whatever he's doing to maintain that body mass and "beer belly" whether it really is drinking beer or eating 5,000 calories per day, the amazing spinning he is doing is not nearly enough to compensate for the volume of calories he's consuming.

Ergo, what he's done is "train his heart" to be super conditioned but at what price. Is his blood pressure through the roof? Does he not profuse blood (poor circulation) to the rest of body thus feeling "cold" all the time? Or does he merely compensate (as is my guess) with a ton of calories much of which are fatty, crappy calories. Remember, simple formula, more out than in. If you're fat ("overweight") you're still taking in too many calories no matter how many you're getting rid of doing spinning or other cardio fitness exercises. My No. 2 example of cardio fit, but not healthy, is almost exactly the same guy as I described above but, in my opinion, a worse example and one you should take note of if you believe in the message I'm trying to convey with this book. The No. 2 example is the guy at my gym who taught karate to dozens of students, including MANY kids weekly. He had the same huge beer belly as my previous reference. The reason this really pissed me off though was because this guy is a third or fourth degree black belt (whatever – I don't know that much about Karate belts – wish I did), and I have no doubt this guy could kick my ass with two fingers and not break a sweat. I do not doubt his level of fitness or ability to kill with his bare hands. What I am disgusted by is his portrayal of a "fit /healthy" image to kids who can look at this guy and say I can be "out of shape," "fat," "overweight," but I can still be a black belt, kick ass, and be a bully. I know I'm taking this to an extreme because I also recognize the fundamental principles of karate, including its respect for the martial arts and that violent confrontation should be the last resort. With that said, and with that understanding, I still believe he's setting a piss-poor example and if your kids are taking karate, or soccer, or any other type of sports training where they are "looking up to a coach," I would strive to find a coach who believes that healthy living should be a message to your kids that's as important as the sport, which they're learning since their chance of going to college or the pros on that sport is about one in 1,000,000.

MY BACKGROUND

I want to paint the picture of myself. I want to focus on Dale the self-proclaimed "fat bastard." I want everyone who's reading this book to understand that I can relate to a piece of them and they can relate to a piece of me. I've had a VERY diverse life and I've tried a ton of things just to say I tried them. **I cannot reinforce the message loudly enough that *if I can do it, anyone can do it.*** Pick the piece or pieces of me that you can relate to and hang onto them. Think about them while you're on the treadmill, elliptical or bike. Let them make you strong, let them make you angry, let them drive you to a better you. You don't have to lose as much as I did, you don't have to get as fit and healthy as I did, but you should, can, and will change your life for the better if you simply follow my basic advice.

The most difficult part about this chapter will be for any of my family who I told to stop reading and who has not yet stopped. I implore you, I beg of you; please skip to the next chapter now. It's going to get ugly and embarrassing and I'm going to admit things that I am not proud of but that are facts of life as a fatty. Am I ashamed of these things that I'm about to discuss? Yes, some of them. Do I regret them? I'd say almost universally, no. I say no because they made me who I am and even if so many people in my life think of me as an asshole than being an asshole it is. I'm healthy, fit, in the best shape of my life and the only thing I fear is getting fat again.

Age

OK, here it goes... Basic statistics: 44 years old as of the time of this book in January of 2014 (I'll be 45 by the time it's published). Caucasian, 5 feet, 10 inch, dark blond short hair, hazel eyes, slim, not Brad Pitt attractive but not Quasimodo either. I was born in June of 1969 in Buffalo, NY. So, already you hate me because I'm a Gemini. Yes, I have two opposite and very distinct personalities. I have a very professional side and a very personal side. They are opposite and its best when they don't converge because like the streams in Ghostbusters™ it's unpredictable what could happen when these two sides meet. I was raised in West Seneca, NY (a small suburb of Buffalo) for the first 18 years of my life. Those years of being raised in a mostly Italian family (75 percent Italian and 25 percent Euro-mutt – dad was 100 percent and mom was 50/50) made me the man I was for 41 years (before I got healthy and stopped some of "the cycle" I was in/on). I was raised "by hand" which in the 70s/80s meant that if I got out of line I got spanked or a hand across the face. Occasionally I got the belt, but I have to admit I didn't get it as much as my four older brothers got it. Yes, I have FOUR older brothers. In 1969, I was the fifth and final pregnancy for my mother. It wasn't until I was 19 and in college that my parents finally admitted that I was a "surprise." Of course, everyone else probably knew since my next older brother is 10 years older than me and my oldest brother is 17 years older than me. My oldest brother was graduating high school before I had my first tooth.

While I had a fairly average childhood, I will go into some of the nuances so that you can relate to some aspect of my life and understand a little more about me. I was an "oops" so when my parents had me my mom was 41 and my dad was 44. Since my brothers were so much older, I was raised as almost an only child to a large extent. By the time I reached an age where I was cognizant of what was going on around me, about 7, I realized that my next oldest brother was almost graduating high school.

Personal Impact

The largest impact on my entire life came when I was 16. This is where it's going to "begin" to get difficult for family members... bail now, pleeeeasssssse! My middle brother was about 28. He and my next oldest brother, who was 26, were still living at home with my parents and I in West Seneca. While I've included my name I'm not going to specifically reference them to protect the "innocent" as much as possible. Part of my parents making up for having me so late in life included yearly trips to Disney World in Florida. We would drive from Buffalo, NY to Orlando, Florida over the course of a couple of days (often taking me out of school for a few extra days at Christmas break). I honestly don't remember the exact year, but I'm going to say it was Christmas of 1984 when we were driving home from Florida. My parents called home while we were driving back up from Florida because my two brothers were able to take care of themselves. They didn't need to come to Florida as they were working or in community college at the time. My one brother told my parents that the other brother had not come home the night before and been gone for a few days.

My brother had "disappeared." The next several weeks (and what seemed like months) were interviews with police, the FBI, and others to file missing person reports. We were all continuously sick with worry. His car had been discovered abandoned in a rest area. Had he been kidnapped, was he doing drugs (it was the 80s), did he "go nuts"? A few weeks later he turned up on my eldest brother's doorstep who, at the time, was living in Florida. My eldest brother gave him some "tough love" and said to get out and straighten himself up. While that was the tough love my parents "probably" would have given him if he had done the same thing to them, it was a critical juncture in my development as that was in effect the last time we heard from him for about 10 years. I really can't appreciate how much this affected my parents and can only imagine how horrible they felt for so long. I can tell you it SIGNIFICANTLY shaped the person I became, both good and bad.

At the ripe age of 16 as an impressionable B- average student, my world was suddenly turned upside down because one of the only two brothers I really knew (the oldest two were out of the house by now) was gone from our lives; and I didn't understand why except for the rumors of drugs or "a girl" or whatever else people theorized. It was about that time that I was deciding what I wanted to be "when I grew up." Was it going to be a career in medicine or computers? Computers were gaming devices to me at the time (funny how that's come almost full circle 30 years later). Medicine would be a difficult long road and I honestly didn't feel I had the grades to realistically succeed. A lack of support by my parents in either direction led me down what I saw as a compromise. After almost finishing this chapter I came back to this previous sentence because I often underplay this point. At one point in my mid-20s one of my parents (I think it was my father) said, "You should turn your hobby into your career and your career into your hobby." This was the best advice they'd ever given; it's a shame they hadn't given it to me 10 years earlier. Being told, "You're not as smart as your brothers and you'll never achieve what they've achieved" was not the motivational/inspirational speech a teenager needed to hear. My hobby at the time will be discussed in detail below.

I would go with computers, but I would also go to the best school I could get into no matter how many loans I had to take out and repay. I was convinced as a big Star Trek fan, at the age of 16 that if I went into computers that the world would be like Star Trek eventually and I would find my lost brother on my own no matter what it took. I had a small Bible that had been given to him for his first communion (yes, I was raised Roman Catholic – more on that later). I still have that small Bible today and as I type it sits on top of my desk. I occasionally flip to a verse even though I'm really not that religious myself (spiritual but not religious – again, more later). Suffice it to say I went to a fantastic university (Rochester Institute of Technology) and got a Bachelor's of Science degree in Computer Science in a five-year program that included a year of co-op experience with IBM in southern NY (Poughkeepsie). I didn't graduate with the best grades in the world but my overall college GPA was about a 3.1. At the time, February 1992, I was dating a woman whom I would eventually move to the Philadelphia area with in 1993 and then get married to in 1995. My wife and I, on my lead, with an "ulterior motive" in my mind would buy into a franchise business that, at the time, pre-Internet breakout, was a technology-based method of "finding long lost relatives" or doing criminal or background checks on individuals for companies or credit checks for apartment renters/landlords. I'm guessing you now see where this is going. We bought the franchise around 1994 or 1995 for about $10,000 and within six months I had already used information I had at my disposal (illegally I might add – I hope the statue of limitations has run out) to find my brother after 10 years. I sent his address to my parents with the caveat that I had obtained it without permission (all of which today is almost silly – a la Facebook and the reverse phone directories – but at the time this was "super secret squirrel stuff" – cut me some slack). They sent him a birthday card for his birthday in February; and to everyone's shock, he called shortly after receiving that birthday card saying that he was embarrassed and ashamed that he hadn't contacted anyone in so long. He said as time went by it got harder and harder because he became more and more ashamed. I think it was probably the single happiest day of my parents' life when he reached back out. This story could be its own chapter, but I'm going to cut it off here because if you were paying attention to what I said and what I didn't say you will understand how this, at the time, justified my last 10 years of existence from the ages of 16 to 25.

Religion

Let's hit an easy, low-hanging aspect of my background that I know MANY of my readers will be able to relate to because it's a common story: Religion. I was raised Catholic, made my first communion, but did not get confirmed until I was in college. I was never really that religious; we'd go to church almost every Sunday (usually dragged along by my father) but never really accepted the whole "gotta have faith" thing. Even at a young age I was always a man/kid of science. Whether it was going to be medicine or computers I went in to, religion didn't have much place in either (from my perspective). When I got to RIT I had a little bit of a spiritual awakening (so I thought – probably, in retrospect, just the stress of college life at a level I didn't feel I was competent to compete at). I got involved in the campus interfaith center and befriended both the Catholic and Episcopal priests on campus. They're views were very liberal for their chosen calling because they understood the connection they needed to make with college kids to get them involved in "church." It was because of this awesome relationship that I began my program of confirmation and eventually became a confirmed Catholic around the age of 20. After I left college I maintained "going to church" for a few years, but I quickly realized what my college priests had shown me was a collegiate approach and attitude to religion and that the rest of the world of religion was never going to "learn" and will eventually, in my opinion, fail for this lack of blind, unwavering, behavior. I am today a spiritual person. I refer to myself as a devout and sometimes militant agnostic. That's kind of a joke – lighten up my born again Christian friends. I firmly believe in karma. I believe in the "golden rule" and I believe this is common to all faiths. I believe that there has got to be something in this universe smarter than we humans are. I believe in the existence of a "higher power" whether that "higher power" is Jesus, Buddha, Allah, men in a spaceship, Wicca, or one of the countless denominations and/or beliefs of any of these faiths. Again, we as humans seem to be too dumb to be the smartest creatures created in the last 100 million years. If this animal that we call human is the best that this "higher power's" got in their arsenal then we're all doomed to blow ourselves up.

Parents' Age

Because my parents were in their 40s when I was born in 1969 you may have already done the math. My father was in World War II in the Army Air Corps (the predecessor to the modern Air Force). My parents were VERY active in their Amvets, VFW, and American Legion posts when I was growing up. I later understood the fraternal reasons to belong to these clubs, besides the cheap alcohol and good parties they often threw. I can't tell you how many German – Polish festivals, pig roasts, or pancake breakfasts I worked at from about 10 – 18 serving pop (soda for those not from western New York) or busing tables and setting up and taking down tables and chairs in dance/catering halls. This was a fairly influential period because I think a lot of the community service I would later do in my life (again, some good and some not so good) came from this upbringing. I don't regret this but looking back on it, it does explain why I eventually had a problem with alcohol (much more on that to come).

The Geek

I mentioned earlier when I was speaking of my brother's story that I was "pretty much" an only child growing up. I need to explain this, I think, because some may be confused how I could be an only child considering I had four older brothers. My brothers were significantly older than me; and while I've been told my whole life that one of my brothers pretty much raised me, I really don't remember it. I will admit that he and I do look almost like twins and have so many similarities (despite our 16 year age difference) that it's hard to doubt we're brothers. My eldest brother was someone I didn't really get to know until later in life; and while I could respect many of the directions and paths he took, he was almost more of a cousin than a brother because I didn't really know that much about him. It's no one's fault, just was what it was. My second brother, similar story to the first, again, not his fault just a fact. I was the ring bearer in his wedding. I know I was probably about 5 or 6 because I'm still mentally scarred from the pistachio green tuxedo with a green ruffled tux shirt I had to wear. VERY 1974! LMFAO... What the hell were you thinking? I know. I've heard since then that it was very spring like and colorful for the time. If I get a picture before I finish this book, I'll publish it.

I knew my other two brothers because they were living in the same house; but remember, if you're in your 40s at this point, how much of the details of your childhood do you vividly remember? I remember a ton of scenarios and scenes, but the timeframes are general and the details fuzzy. Maybe this is because of the years of alcohol, maybe it's because I don't want to remember childhood or anything before the age of 16. Maybe it's my defense mechanism, maybe it's brain cells claimed by Jameson Irish Whiskey that I didn't really need. Maybe it's because I'm always planning for the future and I believe that what's in the past is a "sunk cost" to use an accounting term. I can't recoup what's already spent, so I deal with it., You must decide what investment was positive and what investment was a waste of money.

I know the trips to Disney World and being dragged along to every function with my parents was their attempt to do the best they could while raising me as older parents. They knew they couldn't do some of the things they did with my brothers because by the time I was able to participate in things they were in their 50s; they couldn't afford to chauffer me around to athletics or other extra-curricular activities, so while I was in audio visual class (yeah one of those geeks), or worked on set designs for high school plays, or my brief stint playing the saxophone, I was certainly more of a nerd/geek and would not even be close to a jock (athlete) or a "head" that meant a pot head/druggie at the time. I wasn't a true nerd/geek either because I didn't have the grades to truly be one. So I didn't really fit into a stereotype in high school and that pattern continued when I got to college. I wasn't a nerd, athlete or druggie, so I started drinking because in college you are FREE, so FREE. Too free, but putting on 15 pounds per year (for about four – five years) of college brought me from my high school weight (about what I'm at now – 155 pounds) to my graduating weight of about 210 pounds.

Fraternity

My lack of "fitting in" was also a primary reason that I decided to pledge a fraternity in my junior year of college (yes – you're supposed to do that before you get to be a junior) but I was socially slow/awkward. Pledging also led to my first and only semester (we were actually on the quarter system at the time) of being on academic probation for the 1.75 GPA I got that quarter. Yeah, ouch! That's what happens when you take University Physics III three separate times. I withdrew the first time because I knew I was going to flunk.

Next quarter, I took the same Vietnam-era professor because I felt he was a good teacher and I was just a dumb student. I was wrong. That quarter I got an F. OK, let's take the same class from the Indian professor whom I could barely understand, but had a good reputation. I got a C that quarter and was happy as a pig in poop with a C. Probably also good I became a computer scientist and not a computer engineer. Scientist meant you became someone on the software development or infrastructure side of computers. I choose the former because I really loved programming, seeing the results, and figuring out what wasn't working when it didn't produce the intended results. Hmm, seems this pattern hasn't stopped.

Keyboards/Music

Other tidbits about me you may be able to relate to… So, you think I'm only a geek with a ton of education. You're mostly right. But I am also as right brained. I lean primarily to left-brained thinking, but some amount on the other side (right brained) came from growing up with a Conn Spinet Electronic Organ in our home. When I was on my own, after college, I eventually bought a Yamaha synthesizer, which I owned and played for several years before selling it on Craig's List because I was moving and needed the money to "downsize" my life. I mentioned earlier that I played saxophone for a summer. When my mom told my music teacher that I didn't practice much, they both agreed (no opinion from me) that playing an instrument was probably not for me. In retrospect, I'm really pissed I never learned to play guitar.

50th / Florida

My parents 50th wedding anniversary in 1998 brought my five brothers together in the same room for the first time in about 16 years, most of that time due to my one brother's absence from our lives and the fact that my other brothers all "wisely" left Buffalo as quickly as their new jobs/lives could take them away. Nothing against Buffalo, but it's a classic blue-collar place, and tough to get a professional job. You have to learn to put up with a lot of cold and snow forever. Sorry. Don't worry, I still cheer for the Buffalo Bills whenever they're on TV. Some habits die hard. When I was in my second year of college in 1989, my parents decided I was going to be OK and sold their house in West Seneca. They moved to Florida like so many other retirees. They have lived in Florida since then and as of this writing are still in a house living together and have recently celebrated their 65th wedding anniversary. Since 1998, the five brothers have only been together one more time (for my parents 60th). We're not waiting until the 70th although it's not beyond a reasonable possibility that they could both make it that long. My father's dad died in 1975 at the age of 95 and his mom passed away when she was 99 in the late 1980s. My father's oldest sister just passed away last year (2012) at 100 (almost 101). Super secret… This was a big part of my December 2010 epiphany to get healthy. I have about 50+ years left on this planet and I don't want to be old and out-of-shape and not able to do the things I want to enjoy, IF I ever get to retire.

Family

I mentioned a lot about my family in this chapter – why not – everyone can relate to some aspect of family. What is worth mentioning relative to my lifestyle and being fat was that we were not the closest family, either. We were not a mushy family of "I love you," hugs/kisses, or much "positive reinforcement." Again, you can debate good or bad all day, it just was what it was. I can look back at it now and play Monday morning quarterback and say, "well, if there had been a more supportive environment than maybe things would have turned out better or healthier." Maybe. Maybe not. Receiving a lifetime of negative reinforcement really made the concept of reverse psychology and rebellious behavior a positive motivational message to myself. I was constantly hearing the negative reinforcement so I choose a path of positive self- affirmations that said, "oh yeah, I can't do it, well, I'll prove it." While that concept does work, it isn't without psychological penalties. Did I mention that every ex-girlfriend (and ex-wife) acknowledged what an asshole I am? That many people can't be wrong. And, if I step out of myself I can admit that they're right, but I told them each the same thing. Being an asshole is partially what made me successful and what continues to drive me to succeed. And, might I add, it provides a pretty decent lifestyle because of my choice in computers and senior management.

Career Choice / Move from NY to PA

I said earlier that I chose computers as my field of choice. I really would have made an awesome doctor. I've heard for so many years, "It's not too late; you can still go back to medical school." No, no, really it's too late. A Bachelor's degree in Computer Science and a Master's in Business Administration focused on Management Information Systems / e-Business means that I'd have to do two years of biology and chemistry before I could even take MCAT exams (medical school entrance exams) to get into a two-year MD program and then a four-year internship and then another 4+/- years of residency. In 16 years I'd be... yeah, too late. Start at age 18, finish by the time your 34 and be set for life... That would have been the route. I started in the "real world" after college working at a commercial bank in Buffalo, NY in their Information Systems department as a programmer doing COBOL and Easytrieve™ programming. I did that for a couple years (1992 – 1993) before I choose to follow my college girlfriend to the Philadelphia area because she was moving there for a job, and since I was in computers it was easier for me to get one anywhere. She had the chance to go to North Carolina and while I REALLY wanted her to take that one (weather, golf, and lifestyle) the opportunity in Philly was a better option for her; so I moved to Philadelphia (West Chester, PA) with her. We lived in an apartment in West Chester for about a year until we found a really nice townhouse in the Collegeville, PA area (about 30 miles west of Philadelphia). When I moved to Philadelphia I found another job after a few months doing programming in a language that I'd been transitioning to as I left the bank I was working at.

I was trying to move to PC/Client-Server programming and found a great job doing FoxPro programming. I did that job for a few years until I got "downsized" – which really meant that a new manager was coming on board and wanted to bring in his own people so everyone else had to go. I was out for a couple weeks before I found another similar job programming PowerBuilder and Visual Basic. This time it was for a consulting company and this was the opportunity, three years out of college, which would begin to propel me to the next level of my professional career. For the two years (noticing a pattern?) I was at this consulting company; I moved from programming into quality assurance roles, and then into technical leadership/training roles, and eventually project leadership. Once I had all of this "under my belt" I felt that it was time again to parlay these experiences to the next level of my career. When you're in the information technology field the "vertical market" you're involved in is as important as the technology. I mentioned I started at a bank, and after my move to Philadelphia, worked as a TPA (Third Party Administrator – i.e. insurance related). The consulting company I worked for had many clients; however, I spent a majority of my time at a mutual fund based organization. We see the trend in financial markets so far, right? I'm guessing the theme may continue.

When I was ready to parlay these skills I spoke about earlier, I moved to a large pharmaceutical company in the Collegeville, PA area in 1996 as a project manager. While this was a pharmaceutical company (I know you're wondering about my finance comment a second ago), I was supporting the entire corporate finance function from the CFO to the Controller and every department in between, including Tax, Treasury, A/P, A/R, Consolidations, etc... OK, there's the finance connection. In the late '90s it was a good time to be in the pharmaceutical industry. The industry was producing high-quality amazing medications that returned great revenue, which allowed many of the companies to merge. They knew that this trend would not continue forever. There was a two-year theme going on earlier. Guess what? WRONG! I was at this company for four years until the summer of 2000. I managed the MASSIVE Y2K project for the IT Finance organization and got to travel with our internal audit team to many European countries to assist them with their information systems audits of various pharmaceutical plants and other sales and corporate offices. The reason I took a voluntary exit package exactly four years to the month after I started was because like so many other large pharmaceutical companies they merged with a Kansas City based pharmaceutical company in 1999 – 2000. They were relocating their corporate headquarters from Collegeville, PA to north New Jersey, where I wanted to be about as much as having a hot poker in my eye (well isn't karma a bitch). I had made it all the way up to a Senior Manager at this pharmaceutical company. I took the voluntary package in the summer of 2000 and went to school full-time to finish my MBA through the winter of 2000 and came back into the job market in January of 2001. Guess what, anyone remember the economy and unemployment rates in 2001? That was HORRIBLE timing on my part to decide to "re-enter" the job market. I did another brief consulting gig during the winter/spring of 2001 and finally landed at another Third Party Administration company where I stayed for three years (until February 2004). I went to this new TPA as a Project Manager reporting to a young Manager of Information Technology (IT). I really got into project management at this organization to the point where a good friend of mine, who was actually working for me at this TPA at the time, convinced me that it was time to branch out on my own and be a "real" independent consultant.

DABEL

So, in 2004 I left this TPA and formed DAB Enterprises, LLC. My own corporation was founded on the basis of doing independent consulting specializing in Project Management focused in the Information Technology/ Systems/Services industry. I advertised my specialties as: Project/Program Management, Management Consulting, Imaging / Scanning, Document Management, Application Development, and Solutions Provider. I also listed my areas of focus as: Pharmaceuticals, Financials, Insurance, Healthcare, Manufacturing, "and many others." The friend that had convinced me to join the "dark side" of consulting asked me to work on a large project with him and some of his business partners. That project turned into a nine month +/- effort that parlayed into a few other client engagements. Eventually I ended up working at a pharmaceutical client in Great Valley, PA. I ended up being at this client for about two years before moving on to other clients over the next three years. I worked at another client in Mount Laurel, NJ and then one in Scranton, PA. So, it's worth mentioning for fans of the "The Office" I can say, yes, I worked for a publishing company in Scranton and "there is no party like a Scranton party." During the timeframe from 2004 through 2010 when I worked for "myself" I had very prosperous years and very desolate years. As I've explained to so many people about working for yourself. There are years when you can make $200,000 and years when you make $0. Yes, it evens out in the end as long as you are an expert at managing cash flow.

After six years of working for myself I was looking for a few new things out of my career. This was the longest amount of time I had ever worked for one employer (while the boss was an asshole, he was flexible). I was looking to get back into a corporate environment, I was looking to get back into Senior IT Management, and I was looking to have my own team to manage. As a consultant I missed managing people because one thing I've always been very good at is helping others realize their future potential. In 2010, I found an opportunity with a large generic pharmaceutical company in northern New Jersey. It met all of the criteria I was looking for. It was a large company, I'd be a senior manager in IT (with a good route to Director of IT) and I'd be managing a team (albeit a small team of two people). Making the transition from consulting back into Corporate America was a challenge so this seemed like the perfect opportunity. As with so many other things in my life, "no good deed goes without penalty." While the money and people I worked with were great, I did not anticipate a bi-polar boss who vacillated in between screaming and cursing fits and joking. This was one of my two bosses at the time. My other boss was more of a monotone straight shooter, but I didn't interact with him very often as he was based at the corporate headquarters outside of Pittsburg, PA. My other penalty was I was living on the border of Central New Jersey and North New Jersey and while these are only quasi borders in the state of New Jersey, anyone who's lived in New

Jersey can probably agree that South Jersey should be annexed onto PA because the "south shore" is just an extension of Philadelphia with a slightly different perspective/mentality (more of a relaxed beach culture). Central NJ represented the "most normal" citizens of the state." North Jersey – UGH! All of North Jersey is a bedroom community for New York City and the same attitudes that go with the personality of those who live in New York City. I know I probably have a lot of New York City readers so I'll apologize in advance, but you know you're all a pain as much as I do. You have horrible attitudes, you care about no one but yourself, and everyone else (to you) is an asshole even if you have no basis for that opinion. That's OK; it's just not my personality. So, after my two-year commitment to this company (they paid for my relocation from Pennsylvania) I was already searching for other opportunities. I found a recruiter in Fort Lauderdale, FL that was hot and heavy for talent at a large security company based in Boca Raton, FL. When they called I was like a giddy little girl, "when would you like me there?" I'll take a step backwards and take less money, just get me to Florida. I've been trying to get farther south for 20 years, but between my ex-wife and girlfriends, no one wanted to move to hot and sticky, yucky Florida. So after almost two years of being alone in New Jersey, this was my opportunity to rid myself of the Northeast corridor. Seasonal depression is real and it does not exist when it's not gray and cloudy six months of the year. This two-year period was the beginning, middle, and end of my epiphany about my change in lifestyle and how I got healthy and lost all my weight. I'll go into this more later.

EMS/FF

I have feared this section of the book for a while, so it's somewhat funny to me that it's finally here. This section could easily be its own separate chapter and maybe in future books it will be. As I've been thinking about it over the last several weeks and months I've waffled over whether to go really deep, so everyone can relate to some aspect of this, or just hit the highlights. Like always, there'll be a happy medium. Let me pre-address some foundational statements and apologies I must make before I begin. First and most importantly, I can in all honesty say that I have significantly defined a major portion of my life based on volunteerism and the feeling that giving back to my community is of significant importance to me. I was quoted in my alumni magazine at one point saying: "As someone blessed with more education than one man should have, I feel it's equally as important for people to give back with their time as much as with their money."

When I was growing up my next oldest brother, was a paid EMT and volunteer firefighter. While he was more active at some points in his life than others, he has nonetheless done this "hobby" for 30 years or more. This was certainly my inspiration for getting into EMS (Emergency Medical Services) when I was in college at RIT (my undergrad). My college had an on-campus BLS (Basic Life Support) ambulance that was staffed by an EMT and at least one to two First Aid certified individuals. This meant they had at least ARC (American Red Cross) Advanced First Aid and CPR (Cardio Pulmonary Resuscitation) from either the ARC or the AHA (American Heath Association). I was one of these First Aid individuals. I also became a regular driver of the ambulance and eventually trained other drivers (known at the time as a Driver Trainers, DTs). It was a fantastic experience and really solidified my desire to "give back" and satisfied a need to "help others" when they couldn't help themselves. It also exposed me to a world that I was not familiar with growing up in a lower middle class, blue-collar family in Buffalo, NY. It showed me everything from spoiled rich kids with "quasi" emotional problems (problems we should all be so lucky to have – that is, how to spend mommy and daddy's money) to the darker side of the drug world that again, I had little experience with in my teens/early 20s. The opposite challenge with getting into EMS at such a young age is that the side of life it exposed me to also began what I now reflect back on as the beginning of my narcissistic tendencies. I would not say I have this full-blown disorder, but I can certainly say that my lack of empathy and egotism are directly linked to my chosen hobby.

After I graduated college, I moved back to Buffalo for my first "real" job after college. It was than in 1992 that I got my Instructor certification from the AHA to teach CPR and then subsequently obtained my EMT (Emergency Medical Technician). I was a 23-year-old post-college kid working three jobs, paying back student loans, and trying to have a social life on the side. I worked at my full-time job (programmer at a large commercial bank) from about 7 a.m. until about 4 p.m. I would then run home, change into my EMT uniform and get to the local ambulance company by 6 p.m. to work until 3 a.m. trying to get naps when I could even though we weren't allowed to sleep on the job; however, the benefit of EMS is (similar to law enforcement) your partner always has your back. I would then go home, get a couple more hours of sleep and get back up to do it all over again. On the weekends, at least two times per month, I would go far and wide to teach CPR for the AHA. I can literally say that as an AHA CPR instructor from 1992 until about 2002, I taught thousands and thousands of people the life-saving techniques of CPR and eventually AEDs (automated external defibrillators).

When I moved to Pennsylvania with my girlfriend in late 1993, I applied to the PA Commonwealth Department of Health for reciprocity of my EMT that was granted quickly. I joined a volunteer ambulance service in 1994 (Good Fellowship Ambulance Corps [GFAC] – Station #55) and ran actively with them for about three – four years even after I had moved about 30 miles away to the town I would eventually call home for 15 years. While there are a variety of people that work in the EMS world, and they come in all ages and sizes and levels of experience, I still have a fundamental belief that EMS is primarily a young person's game. Starting at the age I did certainly drove me to a decent level of burn out after about 7 – 10 years. Again, my experience while "running" with GFAC was amazing. I saw the ugly and depraved side of humanity, but I still stuck with my standard quote that I did EMS for stress relief. Many would say, how can you say that job is stress relief? I would always answer the exact same way: "I get stress relief because no matter how bad of a day I think I'm having we roll up on a scene and someone is having a "REAL" bad day. It really helps put your suburban, "white bread" problems into perspective." With GFAC I delivered my first (and to this day only) baby (twins as a matter of fact), but the second baby didn't get delivered until we were putting the mom on the table at the hospital. My partner and I "caught" the first one in the back of our rig on the way to the hospital. It was in that same rig that a year earlier he and I (same partner) would get dispatched to a local doctor's office who had late hours. Men had come in to rob the doctor (a 70+ year old gentleman) for money and pills and shot him in the head. The bullet went through the doctor's left eye and out behind his left ear. It was my job to find the exit wound; but with the blood and gray matter everywhere, I didn't find the exit wound by the time we drove from his office to the helipad waiting to Medi-Evac him to a trauma center; he died a few days later after being in a coma.

Now that I was living in my new hometown (Collegeville, PA), I was getting tired of driving 30 miles each way every other weekend to volunteer for a weekend overnight shift. So I took a leap of faith because at the time I was NOT a "nozzle nut," "fire wacker," "hose head," or "truck guy." In the karma of life I got lucky. The closest volunteer fire company to my new home was a "rescue" company so I didn't have to climb a 150-foot ladder (and while I wasn't scared of heights I was slightly terrified of falling). A "rescue" company, I thought that would be perfect I can still use my EMT skills and slowly get into the "firefighting" side of the business. Thus began 15 years of continuous schooling, education, teaching, and constantly practicing the same skills over and over. Over 15 years, it's no exaggeration to say I sat in thousands of hours of classroom settings and hundreds and hundreds of hours of "live fire" or "live rescue" practice drills. I received certifications in everything from Advanced Vehicle Rescue, to Confined Space Rescue, to Wilderness Firefighting and a Hazardous Materials Technician certification from the EPA (Environmental Protection Agency). There were SEVERAL other certifications over the years. About four years after I joined this local fire company I began to get involved in the administrative side of running the organization. Holy shit, what was I thinking? Anyone reading this right now that's considering doing the same thing, please make sure you're not married, have no kids, no life, and are willing to be a martyr. If all that applies, go for it, otherwise think twice and run away, fast, very fast. I'm only slightly kidding. Around 1999, I began as a "trustee" which meant I was responsible for matters associated with the physical building as well as matters that affected the individuals of the company (disciplinary and the like). I did this for about three years until I eventually became a Vice President and eventually in 2004 the President of the fire company. I mentioned earlier that I am not a very religious man. While I was slightly upset at the time, I cannot tell you much more I believe in karma and have to thank whatever God exists for losing my seat as President in 2010 to the "younger regime" who felt they could do a better job than this "old man." I was 40 at the time. Losing my seat as President propelled me into the next chapter of my life, which enabled my transformation so really; in retrospect, I'm grateful to those who voted against me. Maybe they knew, maybe it was divine intervention, maybe it was karma, maybe it was just time… Either way, it enabled my shift from Collegeville in the spring of 2010 to my new job (back in Corporate America) in northern New Jersey. It was this period, from about March of 2010 until December of 2010 that I was adjusting to my new home and thinking that I was going to be here for at least another five years. It was during this same nine-month period that I was going through some psychological changes and adjustments, which I did not anticipate after being SO entrenched in the firefighting/EMS community for so long. I was breaking up with a girlfriend I had at the time because we used to be an hour apart, which was difficult and now we were about 2.5 hours apart and that made any chance of a "real" relationship almost impossible; and to a large extent I knew (she may or may not have) that I was holding her back just like Collegeville was holding me back. You don't know this when you're intimately involved in the activity, but after you tear yourself away, you realize the "rut" you were in.

Booze

OK, let's tackle the main reason that the fat bastard on the front cover of this book looks the way he does at the ripe old age of 40. The No. 1 reason I looked that way was because I spent a significant portion of the ages between 16 and 40 befuddled, blotto, blitzed, bombed, crocked, dipso, drunk, hammered, juiced, liquored up, pissed, pickled, sauced, smashed, three-sheets-to-the-wind, tanked, and/or shit faced. While I first started experimenting with beer (Genesee Cream Ale) at 16 that included my first vomiting experience from alcohol (but FAR from my last); I didn't really acquire a "taste" for beer until I began my undergraduate college career. They talk about the "freshman 15" which is the 15 pounds you put on when you go away to college in the first year because you're away from home, drinking freely, not exercising (in theory because you're studying), partying more than you should, and eating as you want because, if you paid for the meal plan, it's simply available. I put on the weight associated with the "freshman 15," the "sophomore 10," the "junior 15," the "senior 10," and a special year of co-op education (10 – 20) that was included in my bachelor's degree. I left college about 60 to 70 pounds heavier than when I went in, mostly due to alcohol. Realistically, that went up and down after I left college and because I couldn't "afford" to drink like that anymore since I was repaying student loans and trying to pay for an apartment on my own, and all that life has to offer a college grad who chooses not to go home and live with mom and dad. Between the ages of 23 and 30 my weight vacillated during times of stress or emotional discourse. After my five-year marriage ended in 2000, I was 30 years old and "free again." Free – yeah, what a joke, I was free to try and kill myself with booze and fried food.

AA

What influenced this drinking / indulgent behavior that would eventually, after a few more failed relationships and another eight years, have me attending AA (Alcoholics Anonymous) meetings after a night in a bar almost caused me to shoot someone (literally). I will discuss this later in this book. What I did learn through my AA experience is that each person must decide what the difference between "heavy drinking" versus "alcoholic" means. I have since defined the terms in my own mind, but I have met several other people in "the program" (or similar programs including NA [narcotics], FA [food], SA [sex]) since then who agree or disagree with my interpretation. What most "aholics" will agree to is that there is no way to define someone as an "aholic" if they're not willing to define themselves as one; and equally there's no way to define that you're a "heavy abuser of XXX" versus you are mentally, chemically, physically, and/or psychologically dependant on XXX. Do you need help? HELL YES! Are you an "aholic" of some sort? If you are morbidly fat and unhealthy than I will say, yes you are some type of "aholic." It could be booze, fried food, ice cream, cheese, bread, chocolate, some other food, laziness, chemical, psychological, glandular, a million other reasons. You will conquer it if you listen to my explanations of how I did it and use some, any of my tricks. You are capable of beating your demon. This is a central theory of my belief. We all have our demons and every person's demon is theirs to slay. Some people may think it's one thing but it's really something else. A perfect example is many people only smoke tobacco when they drink alcohol. Which would they define as their demon? Is it the alcohol with its empty calories or the tobacco that inhibits their exercise program? Another example I've had some exposure to (not me personally – I'd say it if I did – there's nothing else I'm holding back in this book) is, "My old demon was heroin, but I'm clean and sober now. Drinking occasional alcohol to excess, smoking cigarettes and a bud of pot per week is OK because I beat heroin." What's their demon? That's a tough one and if you ask 10 people you'll get 15 different answers. If this person was not living a healthy lifestyle, I, Dale, would say their demon is most likely the cigarettes because it's the primary thing in the equation that is inhibiting one of the primary methods of getting healthy (that is, rigorous cardio). But the alcohol – you just said. Yes, but "occasional" was the key word there. The pot gives you munchies. Those munchies can be on fruit or vegetables – I've seen it – not what's dramatized in the movies but possible. The pot may also make them lazy, but if lazy is their demon than the pot merely exacerbates a character flaw; it's not necessarily the reason for the character flaw.

I'll give one last example because I'm notorious for pissing people off so I'll often end sections this way. An obese or morbidly obese teenager who comes home from school, plays video games, eats like crap (fried, fatty food, snacks, sodas, and highly caffeinated beverages) and doesn't participate in gym class at school because they're out smoking with friends or they have a medical note to get out of it because of their obesity. What's this kid's demon? Ready? Oh, I feel the tension rising on this one. Dale's opinion of this kid's demon is the adult piece of shit in their life who allows this behavior to continue because they're feeding their own desire of never having little Johnny or Sarah leave home; and if they're fat and hideous, they'll have to stay home forever so I can be a nurturing mommy/daddy for a long time. And, I as that piece of shit parent, don't set a positive example either because I'm obese and lazy as well. Have you ever heard of it referred to as "the psychological cycle of abuse"? And, many therapists will often be quoted as saying, "you must break the cycle" or "break the chain." I had to break my cycle of drinking and laziness and poor eating habits. It took some of the fundamental concepts I learned in AA and it was far more difficult than getting that way. The negative path is always easier then the positive path but the positive path is so much more worth it in the end. I was raised in a household with parents who were heavy drinkers (not alcoholics – although some may define them as such – I know, now, in retrospect, that they were not alcoholics). Did this influence my behavior? Sure. Was I able to break the cycle? Yes, but it did take me 20 years (50 percent of my life). Am I happier now than I was three years ago? No comparison and saying "yes" understates what getting healthy and having a positive self-image can do for a human being.

LAST TIME, if any family is still reading this chapter, at least I won't have to worry about seeing them at the next family function because if they know I'm coming they won't be there. If they read the rest of this chapter I can also be assured that I'll probably be "unfriended" by them on Facebook, too.

Relationships

I promised myself I would not spend a lot of time on the following subject and thus I will make it only a few sentences long; but in order for a wider audience to be able to relate to me, I must include a brief narrative on my relationships over the last 20 years. As a heterosexual male I can tell you that I've had every experience in relationships that you can imagine, both positive and negative. I have been dating, married, divorced, in long-term relationships (nine years in one case which is longer than I was dating/ married to my only ex-wife). I've had one month relationships (if you can call a one month period of a few dates a relationship). I've dated (and married in one case) an older woman (anywhere from a couple years older to 10 years older). I've dated younger women (anywhere from a couple years younger to 20 years younger). Yes, at 43 I've dated 23. I've dated professional women (lawyer) and I've dated the unemployed and the "blue-collar" women. Some have been educated some have had more life experiences than those with college educations. The only thing that's universally true to this point in my life is that none of these women are still physically with me. All of them are with me in my thoughts and I hope that I'm even with some of them in their thoughts; but as of this chapter I've still not found "the one" I'm destined to grow old(er) with. As promised, I'm not going to go to in-depth in this section to protect the innocent and because honestly it's not pertinent to why YOU need to get healthy, but I did want to give you one more potential area to relate to me on.

This final section of this chapter will deal with a subject where I'm only speaking to the men who are reading this book. As I asked my family to skip the rest of this chapter I will now "offer" that any women (especially those that I've been with) may want to skip the rest of this chapter.

Yes, here comes some of the not too proud moments of my last 20 years. As stated earlier, I won't call them regrets because I don't know that I regret any of them; but they are experiences that have shaped my consciousness and have contributed to my attitude about myself (poorly and positively) and again are an essential part to understanding where I came from when I started this journey.

"Massage"

In the mind of a "fat guy" I was the outwardly happy-go-lucky, funny guy. This was in stark contrast to the "crying on the inside" guy who was so disgusted with his body appearance that when I was introduced to the concept (rather late in life) of massage "happy endings" I was intrigued. I believed in the holistic use of legit therapeutic massage therapy to combat some of issues including low self-esteem and poor self-image. If I could physically "feel better" or have a "release of tension" maybe I could emotionally "feel better." Then, when I found these special massage "therapists" that offered a release that only a guy can appreciate I thought I was dreaming. I knew it was illegal, morally wrong, and the fact that I may have had a girlfriend at the time made it "cheating" on one level, although most guys don't define a physical release as cheating. Ask Bill Clinton. There was no emotional or psychological involvement with these "therapists." It was purely an OK, not great, massage (since none of them are LMTs – Licensed Massage Therapists) that happened to finish in an erotic manner. I honestly looked at it as a favor to my girlfriend at the time because I wasn't "troubling her" to be with a fat, ugly, disgusting mess like me as much as the "horn dog" in me needed the physical stimulation to fill the emotional/psychological void that existed. Well, if you're not completely disgusted by me yet, it gets worse. Maybe you feel sorry for me that I felt I had to go to this level of emotional low to "feel better about myself." Don't feel sorry, I was fat, disgusting, and self-abusive via food, alcohol, and illegal sexual releases.

You've probably heard that marijuana ("pot") is a gateway drug to other drugs. It doesn't matter if you believe that or not, but that you understand what's meant by a "gateway." Some in the drug prevention and medical community will say that drinking alcohol can lead some to smoking more because they only smoke when they drink. Some will say that smoking pot (or poking smot as a girlfriend of mine used to say) will lead you to harder drugs because you want to get higher than you can via pot. Similarly, massages with happy endings were great, but what if I could actually have full out sex with these "therapists." Was that even possible, an option, or would I have to explore new avenues to satisfy my growing desire to be pleasured by women who were unable to make an emotional connection because of the money I was spending on them. Man, did this have a long-term damaging effect on my psychological perspective on dating. It's still having ramifications today. Thankfully Craig's List eventually shut down their "adult" section. Of course, the same site just opened back up under a different name with the same menu of options in any and every major (and not so major) city in the USA. I will not debate drugs any more then I will debate the world's OLDEST profession (mentioned in the Bible), but I state it as a matter of fact about how low my self-esteem as a fat bastard took me. I was willing to risk relationships, my own health (although I was always careful and protected - you just never know), and my future state-of-mind. To this day I get a full blood test every six months and include every sexual test available just to make sure I baseline myself on a regular basis for my own piece of mind as well as any girlfriend I've had since that time. I could probably spend several more pages on this topic of how, when, where, and why I sought out these situations of sexual desire. Many of the women may be reading saying, "all guys are dogs," and this is just a guy being a pervert or a "horn dog" or whatever. Don't lie to yourself piggy. You throw yourself at men at the bar with your fat boobies hanging out hoping to get just one guy's number, hoping to get drunk enough (or get a guy drunk enough) to come home and massage your self-esteem for the evening as well. I've seen it, I've participated in it and I've been told by many women (who will speak with me on the condition of anonymity) that it happens as much as it does the opposite for guys. I will end it with a message to all fatties, men and women. I'm not going to give some "high and mighty" speech about how you should have more self respect and you shouldn't risk the health issues associated with sexually transmitted diseases (STDs); but the reality is that only you will decide when and if you want to address your issues. I hope that you can relate to what I'm saying above and that, as I keep saying, "If fat Dale can do it, so can I." Can you? You're damned right you can. You will. You can. You must.

WHAT INSPIRED ME?

Being fat most of my adult life became the "norm" for me, so arriving at my final epiphany at the age of 41 seems like an odd time for me to arrive at such an obvious point in my life.

Let's talk about the primary influences for getting healthy and "in shape." Any guy (or woman) who tells you ANYTHING other than "being attractive again" is lying (everyone has their own definition of attractive but what I GUARENTEE is that attractive, in every case, means NOT obese). I know what you're thinking. He got skinny for "poon tang"? REALLY? Yes, you want honesty or you want it sugar-coated? Again, male or female, straight or gay, it doesn't matter. You're getting healthy and as a result you will be more attractive to yourself and to others. You may not envision yourself as a Ken doll or a Barbie or a J Lo, Angelina Jolie, Brad Pitt, George Clooney, or Matt Damon, but I can guarantee that attractive almost never means the physical appearance of Roseanne Barr, Aretha Franklin, Rosie O'Donnell, Joseph R Gannascoll (think Soprano's Johnny Cakes), Sally Struthers, Steven Segal (later years), John Candy, Artie Lange, Honey Boo Boo, and Vincent Pastore (Soprano's "Big Pussy"). The list is long and you do not have to agree with me, but if you think that anything in our society promotes "fat" or "obese" as "sexy" than you may not be at the mental low point you need to be in order to follow my advice. You should probably go back to chapter one and start the book over. Seriously, fat is disgusting. You can control yourself. You may not want to but the more results you see the more you will be pissed at yourself for waiting this long and not doing anything about it. Granted, if you're too old to care anymore than maybe this book was a waste of your time and money (no refunds – give it to your fat kids or grandkids). However, be cautious if you say, "I'm too old." You may think/feel that but the person you're still with may not. If that person has been with you for some ungodly number of years (defined in my book as more than one) than maybe you should rethink that statement.

Duh

So yes, being more physically attractive and the desire to increase my likelihood of obtaining a more attractive selection of women than I previously dated was a primary influence. Before all my ex's get too pissed and start sending me threatening text messages... It's worth pointing out that I didn't date ugly women just women that were "appropriate" considering my level of physical attractiveness. OK, that wasn't much better but I still say the women I was with were NOT piggly wigglies. When I got healthy and more self confident, I naturally projected a very different front and naturally attracted a different type of person. We are a pack mentality species. We navigate towards others like ourselves in whatever manner that means. It could be age, race, religion, sex, and yes, often size.

Let's define physically attractive. Beauty is in the eye of the beholder, but ugly goes clear to the bone. Sure, our modern era of television has shaped the reality of our culture. However, for the purposes of this book I'd like to draw a clear distinction between what is considered "healthy" and "obese". See non-scientific chart below to determine "Healthy" versus "Not Healthy". Which one are you closer to? If I were to go back in time (50 – 60 years) I could easily show pictures of Marilyn Monroe, Cary Grant, and Frank Sinatra and while they may not have been as "svelte" as our modern celebs they're still a contrast to Abbott and Costello, Raymond Burr ("Ironsides" – sorry the beard didn't hide the second or third chin), or Chubby Checker.

I must comment on the table below. It would be a travesty of my soul if I did not mention it. I've mentioned a few times in this book that the lawyers would eventually catch up with me. God damn pricks! The table below had pictures of the celebs I wanted to showcase as being "healthy" versus "unhealthy" but a small clause called, "for editorial use only" screwed me after I already paid for what I was led to believe was the right to use these photos in the publishing of my book. So, instead, I've described the images; however I would encourage you to Google the text I've included to see the actual pictures I'm referring to within this table.

Healthy:	Two classic actors – both middle aged but defined as handsome, physically in shape, always dressed well in tailored custom European cut suits. Google the following phrase for the pics: Brad Pitt & George Clooney at hand & footprint ceremony at Grauman's Chinese Theatre for the stars of "Ocean's Thirteen." June 5, 2007 Los Angeles, CA	One of the Charmed Ones – in so many ways. She has always been a personal favorite and has matured over the years into an amazing beauty with a slim figure and flowing brunette hair often seen in her skinny jeans. Google the following phrase for the pics:Actress ALYSSA MILANO at the Los Angeles premiere of Monster in Law. April 29, 2005 Los Angeles, CA. 2005	Beauty and sexuality combined into one. Angelina Jolie is so healthy that she voluntarily underwent a double mastectomy to avoid the eventuality of breast cancer. That takes a healthy lifestyle to a new level. Google the following phrase for the pics: LOS ANGELES, CA - JULY 19, 2010: Angelina Jolie at the premiere of her new movie "Salt" at Grauman's Chinese Theatre, Hollywood.

Healthy:	One of the funniest, most under-rated comedians of this generation. Jim Norton has been a masterful talent for Jay Leno and Opie and Anthony. He is the self-proclaimed "calf kid". He has calves of steel from his massive amount of elliptical work. You go little Yimmy. Google the following phrase for the pics: NEW YORK-OCT 3: Comedian Jim Norton attends 'Everything Or Nothing: The Untold Story Of 007' premiere at the Museum of Modern Art on October 3, 2012 in NY City	Speaking to my early comments about, no excuses, I've often heard from black friends that it's more difficult for those of non-Caucasian races to maintain a healthy lifestyle. Again, I say, bullshit. Kerry Washington shows this healthy living as an art form. Google the following phrase for the pics: Kerry Washington at the 24th Annual Producers Guild Awards, Beverly Hilton, Beverly Hills, CA 01-26-13	Similar to Kerry Washington a brilliant example of a man maintaining the same healthy living is Will Smith. Google the following phrase for the pics: Actor Will Smith attends the screening of RAISING HELEN at the Tribeca Performing Arts Center for the 2004 Tribeca Film Festival May 1, 2004 in New York City	Charlize Theron showing that you can import someone from another country (South Africa) and maintain a healthy lifestyle even after indulging in the American pastime of overabundance. Google the following phrase for the pics: Charlize Theron at the 69th Golden Globe Awards at the Beverly Hilton Hotel. January 15, 2012 Beverly Hills, CA

Not Healthy:	Artie Lane is the opposite picture of Jim Norton above. While few can debate Artie's comedy anyone that knows his unhealthy history knows that recovery from addiction is not easy and while I wish Artie was physically healthier he shows the antithesis of Mr. Norton above. Google the following phrase for the pics: STUDIO CITY, CA - AUGUST 13: Artie Lange at "Comedy Central's Roast of William Shatner." August 13, 2006 in CBS Studio Center, Studio City, CA.	Aretha Franklin may be one of the greatest singers of her generation but her weight issues are no mystery to anyone that has sight. Google the following phrase for the pics: Aretha Franklin at the Sony BMG Music Entertainment party at the Beverly Hills Hotel following the 2008 Grammy Awards. February 10, 2008 Los Angeles, CA	The man who wants to become President of the United States. It's rumored that he's recently gotten stomach surgery. While I surely hope he is doing something and while I don't endorse the surgery because I believe he can control it himself I think he would set a horrible example to be the fattest President since Taft. This obesity would be a horrible example for Americans and a joke of a picture to the rest of the world about America's gluttony issue. Google the following phrase for the pics: WESTFIELD, NJ- FEBRUARY 8: New Jersey Governor Chris Christie continued his "New Jersey Comeback" theme at a town hall meeting held at the Westfield Armory located in Westfield, N.J. on February 8, 2012.	Someone who prides themselves on their obesity and feels she is an example of a voluptuous woman. Sorry, Rosie O'Donnell, fatness and the acceptance of it is just a poor example for young women. Google the following phrase for the pics: HOLLYWOOD - AUGUST 25: Rosie O'Donnell at the "Nip Tuck" Season Four Premiere Screening at Paramount Pictures on August 25, 2006 in Hollywood, CA.

In December of 2010 I went on vacation to surprise my parents who were spending Christmas with my eldest brother's family in Tennessee. I had already planned on flying right from Nashville (my brother's home) to Key West after Christmas to spend New Year's there, by myself to have a "man-cation" and be alone and contemplate my life changes over the last year of moving to New Jersey. Through a series of events it was here that I had my grand epiphany. There were a number of factors that brought me to this low point in my life, but the forces of the universe aligned to bring me to the emotional low where I needed to be in order to enable my "great transformation." There were 41 years of experiences leading up to this grand epiphany, but I will list the two straws that "broke the camel's back."

In November of 2010 while I knew I was going to Nashville and Key West, FL for the holidays I went in to get my annual blood test results from my doctor. I purposely went to see a short fat Italian doctor because I always felt like I could say, "Yeah? I have to lose weight and exercise more? Are you the pot or the kettle doc?" But this visit was different. I'd been used to all of my numbers being "off the charts" for years. Blood pressure, cholesterol, triglycerides, sodium, and every other bad blood test result you can have. We had a family history of all these things. I knew I was eventually going to have to be on Lipitor®. I knew I was going to have a heart attack eventually. It was like a rite of passage in my family. What threw me for a loop was when my doctor said, "Your liver enzymes are off the charts." I said, in my usual smartass manner, "OK, how much can a liver transplant be"? He said, "It costs $750,000 and it's not covered because you're an alcoholic." I said, "Fuck you, I'm not an alcoholic, I can slow down or stop drinking any time I want. I choose not to – I'm not a quitter!" He said, "No, you're probably not an alcoholic but you are certainly a binge drinker and you must cut back or you are going to do permanent, irreversible damage to your liver." I said, "No, screw you, I will stop." He repeated, "You don't have to stop, you need to back off." Well, anyone who knows me knows that I typically don't do many things half ass. Thanks OCD! I reflected on this conversation while I went to Nashville the following month and Key West for New Years. While I was contemplating whether or not I really wanted to stop drinking while I was in Key West, I had an experience at one of my favorite bars in Key West (the Garden of Eden) that would be the final nail in this coffin.

While sitting at the bar a day or two before New Year's I was wearing my niece's fire company t-shirt (she is my brother's daughter from Nashville). Yes, many within my family got into the volunteer EMS and firefighting community eventually. Anyway, I was wearing her company's t-shirt while I was sitting at the Garden of Eden bar. If you haven't gone to Google yet you'll soon discover that the Garden of Eden is the only "clothing optional" bar in Key West. There was a woman and her husband at the end of the bar tying a load on and we got into a friendly discussion about "are you a firefighter"? I was going through, explaining yes I was a volunteer firefighter, but this was my niece's company in Nashville. The woman said, "I'd love to have that shirt, I collect fire company shirts." My niece is going to kill me – she better not be reading this. I took off my shirt since clothing wasn't required in this bar anyway and tossed it across the bar to her. She thanked me and then leaned over and started whispering to her husband. I suddenly realized it was fairly cold on this particular night. The next thing I heard was her and her husband giggling and she pointed over at me and all I heard her say was, "Oh my God, look at those bitch tits." In my usual fat bastard mind I laughed and said to her, "you're just jealous." Timing is everything in life and this woman (I can't even call her the horrible name I want to call her) nailed it. It was a perfect shot at me. I had to walk downstairs a few minutes later because it was so damned cold that I had to buy a t-shirt on the street. Fortunately, I found and bought a XXL Garden of Eden t-shirt that I had until recently when I finally gave it to Goodwill. It was a reminder of where I came from but now, only three years later it seems like such a distant memory that I needed to rid myself of this horrible reminder of such an unhealthy time in my life. While sitting in the hot tub over the next few days at my hotel the revelation came. This was it; I was going to do it. I couldn't believe I was saying it or even that I could really do it. January 1, 2011 was the last time I drank ANY alcohol for the next five months. This will be examined more in some upcoming pages.

Blood Work

So, let's talk blood work. I've included a listing of the numbers below including the before and after. As I said in previous pages, I'm not a doctor (I couldn't get enough positive reinforcement/encouragement when I was a youngster for that) but I can tell you what it means for your total cholesterol and your LDL cholesterol to be sick high (253). I can tell you that having triglycerides in the high 200's (290) when they're supposed to be below 150 is bad. I can tell that a liver enzyme score (abbreviated as GGT on your blood test results – related to the ALT/AST test) should be between nine and 60 and while mine is currently in the neighborhood of 30 it peaked in November of 2010 around 108. This is when the doctor and I argued about my status as an alcoholic. Five months without booze and only returning to two glasses of wine (maximum) per week helped reduce this score under 60 within nine months. This removal of alcohol also helped the triglycerides go down to about 80 (less than 150 is good) from a score of 290.

The chart below shows the numbers four months after I began my plan of "healthy living" versus the "three months before" picture that is handwritten by my doctor next to the updated numbers. Not a bad reduction for four months. It only got better with time and the numbers on the rest of the blood work also continued to improve.

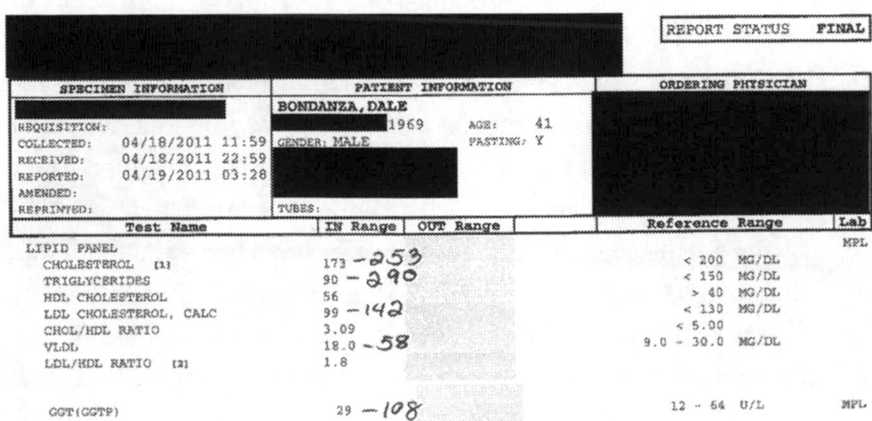

REPORT STATUS FINAL

SPECIMEN INFORMATION	PATIENT INFORMATION	ORDERING PHYSICIAN
REQUISITION:	BONDANZA, DALE	
COLLECTED: 04/18/2011 11:59	1969 AGE: 41	
RECEIVED: 04/18/2011 22:59	GENDER: MALE FASTING: Y	
REPORTED: 04/19/2011 03:28		
AMENDED:		
REPRINTED:	TUBES:	

Test Name	IN Range	OUT Range	Reference Range	Lab
LIPID PANEL				MPL
CHOLESTEROL [1]	173 – 253		< 200 MG/DL	
TRIGLYCERIDES	90 – 290		< 150 MG/DL	
HDL CHOLESTEROL	56		> 40 MG/DL	
LDL CHOLESTEROL, CALC	99 – 142		< 130 MG/DL	
CHOL/HDL RATIO	3.09		< 5.00	
VLDL	18.0 – 58		9.0 – 30.0 MG/DL	
LDL/HDL RATIO [2]	1.8			
GGT(GGTP)	29 – 108		12 – 64 U/L	MPL

What else inspired me? I mentioned the obvious right off the bat…it's puss, puss. Again, I'm a red-blooded, heterosexual male with a new body and an increased level of testosterone from all of the healthy living and exercise. Why shouldn't I enjoy the benefits of this level of testosterone that I haven't seen since I was 18 years old? Except, now that I'm in my 40s, I don't have the "quick draw" trigger of an 18 year old. So, let's talk about the effects of testosterone on the body (male or female). Most of us know the usual things that come along with testosterone versus estrogen. Testosterone makes your muscles stronger, makes you grow hair, makes you more assertive/aggressive (focus on the assertive part) and assists in sexual relations. Yes, this all applies for both sexes. While women don't generally appreciate the increased hair in sensitive places it's a small price to pay for the healthy benefits of exercise. Estrogen, however, is the ultimate poison for a man (and while women can't live without it, an excessive amount due to FAT is not good either). You've heard of "too much of a good thing," right? Women know that as they age, into their 40s, 50' and beyond that they slowly lose the "estrogen advantage" that reduces their cardiovascular risk until this age. Ergo, once their estrogen starts to decline (indicative of moving beyond child bearing) their levels of testosterone actually rise because they're not being restricted by the estrogen anymore, which again can make women more physically competitive as they grow older. Can you imagine that? Women – if you started exercising now (especially if you're 40+) you can actually get stronger and faster than the 30-year-old version of yourself (age graded of course). Why did I say estrogen is a poison for men? Both men and women have both testosterone and estrogen in differing percentages. In general, and for normal, healthy people, men's proportion of testosterone outweigh women's levels; and women's levels of estrogen outweigh men's levels. That's easy enough. What do excessive levels of estrogen in men cause? You may have heard me mention my low point earlier. Do a search in this text for the words "bitch tits." High levels of estrogen can also lead to prostate cancer, loss of erectile strength and libido. Excessively obese men have very high levels of estrogen. This will increase your body fat percentage (bitch tits), allow for excessive belly fat (beer belly/gut), make you more emotional and sensitive (less assertive/aggressive), increased risk of diabetes, increased risk of cardiovascular disease, hair loss, and the obvious, overall reduction in the amount of testosterone. So, this is why I consider estrogen to be a poison for men.

Suffice it to say that there were sexual benefits I experienced from getting healthy, lowering my resting heart rate to the 50s (less than one beat per minute) and lowering my blood pressure to near double digits on top (systolic) and in the 60s/70s on the lower end (diastolic). The ability to maintain arousal, erection, and go for hours at a time are normal side benefits of getting healthy. Did I mention earlier the increased length of your penis from weight loss? Guys, do you know it's been proven that for every 35 pounds of fat that you lose you gain an inch on your penis? Yes, I lost more than 70 pounds so I can testify that it's true. It's not just penetration depth because you have less fatty deposits around your belly and hips, its actual length. I can attest to formerly (the fat Dale) being typically "average" in length. I can attest to the healthy Dale being "above average." I'm still not John Holmes; but I can confidently say, I'm much happier with my new self image.

I mentioned my blood test results earlier. Another benefit of getting healthy is the ability to look at blood test results and not just smile but openly laugh. To think that I was close to biological death with my previous numbers makes me look at my cholesterol, glucose, AST/ALT, scores and think how in such a short time I could make such a fundamental shift in my life and health. Reviewing these results so many times has also made me a bit of an expert in these numbers; so now when friends say, "Hey Dale, can you look at my blood work and tell me if my doctor is telling me to do something that I don't really need to do." I can tell you that most doctors won't tell you to do something because it benefits them. They are often, however, reacting to what they're reading on a piece of paper. "Your cholesterol's high!" Take Lipitor, Crestor, or other cholesterol- lowering meds. Eat less meat, exercise more, and take fish oil. There's a reason they spent 12 – 15 years in college; they're a lot smarter than you and me. They are, however, still human beings. They are not "all knowing." They do not know how your body will react to different things (drugs, exercise, natural vitamins, etc…). They can take a reasonable guess based on what they've learned and other statistics, but at the end of the day there's a reason it's called "practicing medicine."

Another small observation I've made over the course of my professional career in the Information Technology field. I've extended this observation beyond the realms of geeks into other areas like Finance, Accounting, Human Resources, Marketing, Sales, etc... Look at the ranks of management from first line supervisors to managers, directors, vice presidents, presidents, and C level executives. On average, no statistics to back me up, although I bet I could find some. The majority of these managers are NOT obese or morbidly obese (see our earlier definitions of those conditions). They may have a couple extra pounds (making them technically fat), but that doesn't necessarily qualify them as obese. If you were putting in those numbers of hours and giving up hours after work and on the weekends and taking time away from your family, you may have more difficulty maintaining a good diet as well. The funny dynamic that I've learned about getting healthy is that when you look better and feel better about yourself that heightened self-esteem translates to more self-confidence; thus, it makes you more successful in your boss's eyes and thus more promotable. Other obvious things to consider include that people want to work for more attractive people. There's a natural quality that someone who knows their business and is in shape/attractive adds to their leadership style. They inspire more; they speak about doing 5Ks or triathlons, or bike races. They inspire people, they don't talk about the "all you can eat Chinese buffet they went to this weekend and gorged themselves until they had to un-button their pants." You may work for either of these types of bosses, but I can tell you although some people would resent the "more attractive manager/boss" they'd rather work for them then "Slob-o."

While I can't say that doing better at sports actually inspired me to get healthy, and the converse is certainly true. I didn't aspire to get better at sports, but I certainly didn't want to continue to suck at everything I did from volleyball to my hobby of firefighting. I'd say years of being in firefighting as a "volunteer" always disturbed me because if there's a hobby that you should do AND be healthy this would be the one. Yet, more often than not volunteer firefighters are minimally fat and typically obese or worse. It bothers me that I didn't choose to get healthy until I was no longer an active volunteer. A part of my "recovery" from obesity is that I want to give advice and inspiration and words of encouragement to all that do any type of public safety as a hobby or a profession. You CANNOT serve and protect if you CANNOT serve and protect your own body. The reason this particular paragraph was difficult for me to write is because I've been so obese most of my life, it's hard to refer to myself as an athlete. I was on a date recently and I was explaining my "hobby" of running and the woman asked me if I was competitive. I said, "All runners are competitive. Most, including myself, are competitive with ourselves." But, in all reality I really am "somewhat" competitive within my age group and what amazes me is that I will continue to get faster as I get older. This formula has been explained to me by senior runners and coaches and as I continue to train and do my once a week "speed work."

My final inspiration, in more than one sense, is my personal "bucket list." It's definitely cliché at this point to refer to one's own bucket list but I will admit under my Gemini "personal side" that I'm an "emo" with sad movies. Like many who saw the movie "Bucket List" with Jack Nicolson and Morgan Freeman, I was affected by its message. The movie itself was the typical Hollywood crap about the dumb rich white guy and the poor super intelligent black guy; and how the man with nothing could teach the man with everything more than he ever learned in "school" or in "business." Despite the overall typical sub-standard plot line the movie spoke to subtleties in my own life that rightfully got me to make a list. It helped me out of the depression I was in at the time because it let me know that there were some definitive things I didn't want to leave this earth without doing. One of the items on the list was "to be satisfied with the way I look." It was seemingly innocent when I put it on the list. (My list was created the same year the movie first came out.) I had no idea how this goal would be satisfied. Would I finally just accept my obesity? Would I see a plastic surgeon? Would some divine miracle occur? I'm fairly certain that getting healthy in my eating and exercise habits was not what I was thinking at the time. Some of the goals on my list were purely self-serving (just like in the movie). Some of my goals were more altruistic. Some will probably not truly be achievable in my remaining years on this planet.

MY PLAN

"Nobody ever wrote down a plan to be broke, fat, lazy, or stupid. Those things are what happen when you don't have a plan."

"Don't worry about the failures, worry about the chances you miss when you don't even try."

"When you say 'it's hard,' it actually means "I'm not strong enough to fight for it." Stop saying it's hard. Think positive!"

After my epiphany in December of 2010/January 2011, I returned to northern New Jersey where I was living at the time (Hillsborough, NJ) with a secret mission that only I knew. I would keep to myself for about two months until my mission started to appear obvious to those around me. I already belonged to the local gym (Hillsborough Racquet and Fitness Club (HRC) – free plug). At least two of the participants from the hit TV show "Biggest Loser" worked out at this same gym as well. While, at the end of the day, I personally lost a higher percentage of total body weight than the guys that appeared on the show, I did not start at the obesity level that they started at so their total loss compared to mine (raw pounds) was significantly more than me. I found a dietician in the town of Somerset who was referred to me through my health plan at the time. Her cost was not covered by my health plan but at the time, that didn't matter to me because… "I was on a mission." There were two personal trainers (PTs) at the HRC. There was a male and a female and I choose to work out with the guy because his hours were more aligned with my availability. At the time, that was about the only criteria I used since there were only two trainers at the club that I had to choose from.

Before I get into the specifics about my dietician and my PT, I need to preface it with my first approach to losing the weight. I was morbidly obese (by percentage over ideal BMI) and I knew that once I reached this level I was technically eligible for the lap band or stomach stapling because as our country's mentality believes it is better to offer slobs the "easy out" because it will save us all money in the long run by helping offset future co-morbid conditions of obesity. Since the obese are more likely to suffer from diabetes, cardiovascular disease, high blood pressure, and many other disorders, it is cheaper to allow the disgusting, pathetic, "I can't make my own right choices" the ability to choose the cheaper, easier out. Surgery absolutely comes with risks. You can die while under the knife or due to complications. Of course, you can die stepping off the street corner, going to a movie theater in Colorado, or going to school in Lancaster, Pennsylvania no matter how devout of a religious zealot you think you are. You can certainly die on a treadmill, running on the street, on a bike (in the gym or on the street), swimming in the pool or open water, but death will certainly come to all of us eventually. You are more in control of the "when" than you think.

Plastic Surgeon

I went to see a plastic surgeon in Morristown, New Jersey in August of 2010 just outside of the five Boroughs of New York City. I will give him the free plug because he was awesome, friendly, and told me exactly what I didn't want to hear. Maybe because I'm such a realist I think that's so rare; but he was really professional about telling me what I needed to know. His name is Dr. Brian S Glatt MD, FASC. I'm sure my lawyers/editors will make sure I get his release before posting his name in my book. If his name is here and you're in northern New Jersey I highly recommend him. If his name didn't make my book then he wouldn't sign the release form so to heck with him. Kidding, he still did right by me, big time. So, I took a half of a day off of work to go see this doctor in his office. Why would he have weekend hours? He's a ludicrous millionaire from making beautiful boobies, tummy tucks, and liposuctions. The fat bastard on the cover of this book, the one with "bitch tits" went in having done my usual ton of Internet research saying OK, I know I need abdominal liposuction, male breast reduction, and probably liposuction from my neck and possibly a corresponding neck tuck/face lift. I knew the total procedure would probably be in the $10,000 - $20,000 range and completely uncovered by health insurance. He came in and actually "talked to me." Imagine that shit! He spent the better part of 30 minutes with me. He took pictures from every angle. He squeezed, poked, and prodded all of my fat and said, "give me a few minutes" and "let me analyze what we have here and I'll come back in and we can talk." I waited in nervous anticipation thinking about everything I had read online about hospital charges being separate from anesthesia charges, and how long the recovery process would be after the surgery. I was over concerned about the scar that I would have across my pubic region from one side of my waist to the other almost looking like a belt. How long would I be black and blue? If I got rid of my gut would I be able to finally start working out and get six-pack abs? I read that once you have liposuction the fat cells in those areas sucked out and NEVER come back; but if you continue to live a horrible diet fat will come back in other places that were not treated. I thought *what if I get male breast reduction and all of a sudden I start getting fat under where my man boobs were? What if I developed side boobs?* Hell, while we're taking all the fat out of my ass doc can we put some in my manhood to at least give me something to show for all this money? I was nonetheless confident that with the possibility of him taking 20 – 30 pounds of fat thus I would easily be on my way to be able to start to lose the weight on my own, but I needed this stimulus to get me there.

Dr. Glatt came back into the room, sat down and laid out exactly what he could do. He had me once again pull my hospital gown aside and pinched the fat from my belly. He methodically explained that the amount of fat and skin he could take off of me amounted to about five – seven pounds. I'm shocked and stunned. He's still pinching my belly (kind of starting to hurt) and he says, why do you think I can't pull any more fat then this? He explains that my fat is visceral fat not subcutaneous fat. Visceral fat is the fat that develops underneath the muscle not under the skin as is the case with subcutaneous. Think of the skin as your outside protective shield. Under the skin everyone has some layer of fat. Under the fat there is muscle. Under the muscle are all of the internal organs, bones, and innards. Keeping this simple – this ain't a medical book. ☺ If you develop fat between the muscle and internal organs it's called visceral fat. Dr. Glatt explained that in order to remove the five – seven pounds of subcutaneous fat would cost me around $8,000; but at the end of the day I wouldn't be happy because he's not going to be able to sculpt me the way I want to be sculpted. He said point blank, "take half of the money you were going to give me, go get a personal trainer, and come back and see me in six months and then I'll help you out and you'll be much more satisfied." Wow, was that a slap in the face for the 40 hours of Internet research I did studying about every type of liposuction in the world and the effects, recovery, costs, side effects, etc… would be. The consultation visit cost me $100 but I think it was the best $100 I ever spent on my road to getting healthy. For a doctor to tell me there was nothing he could do to make me happy and that the only way to get rid of this visceral fat was cardio, cardio, cardio (his words), I was half excited but equally depressed. This was NOT the answer I was hoping for but one I should have probably expected.

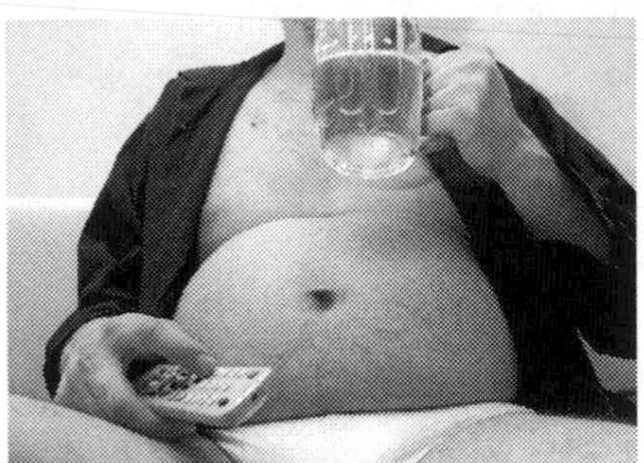

Visceral Fat (the famous beer belly)

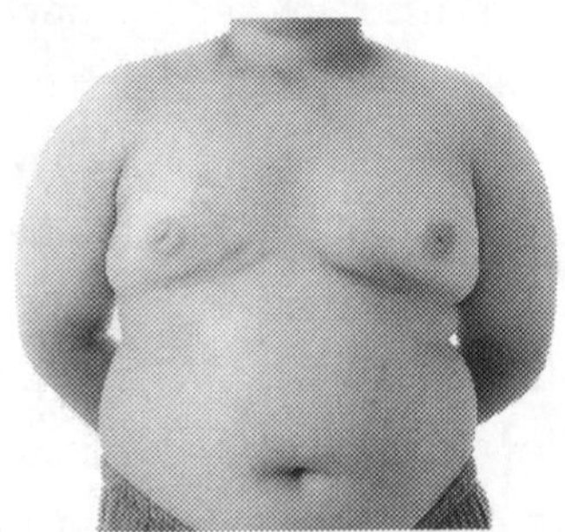

Subcutaneous fat and parents who should be shot

The timing of everything in this chapter is important for you to understand. As I write it and look back over the time period, my knee jerk reaction is that it took longer to come to this realization than even I thought; but, in fact, I will say Dr. Glatt's visit in August of 2010 was the point in the roller coaster just before you reach the top of the first hill. It was not the "straw that broke the camel's back," but it was a pretty big weight on my shoulders. I was fully prepared to spend $15,000 on plastic surgery even though I was sickened by the thought of a fat solution like gastric bypass or the lap band.

Two months after my experience with Dr. Glatt is when I went to my regular doctor for my annual blood test, which I've always been strict about since my early days as an EMT. I was taught early on in my EMS career that it's always good to have an annual (or more often) baseline. Then, as I began to live the "lifestyle" of a degenerate, fat, loser I knew it was even more important to get a regular baseline. This visit in October of 2010 is the one I describe in detail in the previous chapter. Four episodes, each two months a part, means more when I look back at it than it did at the time. I joined my local gym in June of 2010. Then I had my visit with Dr. Glatt in August. Then, after my visit with my regular doctor in October, and then came my Christmas (December) holiday visit with the family followed by my "man"-cation in Key West post-Christmas through New Years. Seven to eight months from June of 2010 (my 41st birthday) until January of 2011.

I had belonged to my local gym in New Jersey since June of 2010 (where I was living in 2010/2011), but I joined it primarily because it was close to my apartment and they had racquetball courts. I loved playing racquetball when I was younger and thought this might be a good way to get me inspired to start working out more regularly. Besides, there were other fat guys who played racquetball, so it must be a "sport" a fat guy can be good at. I played in the leagues at the club for three seasons before I realized I wasn't getting any better and was consistently being beaten by men twice my age (almost) one of which used an inhaler often during our match. I thought this was an unfair advantage. "Hey old man, pass out the corticosteroids to everyone."

Similar lesson to one I'd learn about Yoga… Over time, anyone can get good at anything. Healthy living, diet and exercise are all great examples of this.

I need to explain my 11 months in the 12-step program of AA (Alcoholics Anonymous) to clear the air and allow others to relate to my challenges and situation. I spent two stints in "the program." My first experience was from September of 2008 until February of 2009, and my second was from January of 2011 (the beginning of my new Healthy journey) until June of 2011. I owned my own company doing consulting in the Information Technology field surrounding Project Management. Remember 2009 was a rough year in the economy (they'd all been but 2009/2010 were particularly difficult in my area). My last paycheck in 2009 from the company I was working for came in April of 2009. In case you're not familiar with the "white-collar world" and especially Information Technology, finishing an assignment on the precipice of summer is about the worst possible time you can finish an assignment. I looked, I offered, I wrote proposals for projects but nothing was coming to fruition. I did what I always did during lapses or during "bench time" as we called it in the business. I continued to live my life as if the next gig was right around the corner.

What I didn't realize is that my drinking would increase, significantly, as I felt more depressed about not working and not having an income coming in. I had my house on the market because I also knew after a recent breakup with my girlfriend of eight-plus years (that's a whole different book) that I needed to downsize and was fully prepared to move back into an apartment. I had liquidated a significant portion of my house assets for pennies on the dollar via Craig's List and gotten myself down to the point where I knew I could fit comfortably into an 800 square foot apartment after spending the last nine years in a 2,200 square foot home that was packed with crap. By August of 2009 when I hadn't had many leads on the house, no prospect of a job on the horizon, savings being spent like water, and booze going down the hatch like I was trying to drink myself to death (hmmm… ya think?), it came to the point that it only has one other time in 41 years; it caused me to completely lose my mind. Similar to a blackout drunken episode, except mine was rage.

I became so enraged at the bar on some random night in August of 2009 about my lack of future, I was literally at the point of murdering another human being because unbeknownst to him he was the poor unfortunate slob who happened to flip my switch that night. I don't just mean I was going to beat the daylights out of someone in a drunken, retard display of strength. I was a concealed carry permit holder in Pennsylvania and unlike other states that wisely don't allow you to carry your firearm into a bar, PA's not got that one down yet. I know there is a Higher Power and I know "some portion of my upbringing" must have resonated enough with me not to pull my Kel-Tec 9mm and end my pain at the time; only to start a new pain of which I would never recover. That was enough of a "bottom" for me. Yeah, that's my "bottom." "So," I said when I woke/sobered up the next morning, "maybe it's really time to consider that AA thing." Friggin' rocket scientist I was, huh? September of 2009 saw my first AA meeting near my hometown of Collegeville.

Guess what fans? Do you know what being sober gets you? To quote a movie line it allows you to "unfuck your mind." There were pros and cons to my turbo sobriety. Retrospectively, it turned out more cons than pros. Things came together for me sooooo quickly once I stopped drinking. I was able to get my head around selling my home and moving into an apartment in the same town where I'd spent 15 of the last 17 years at the time. I went to networking events and met old colleagues who knew of my work situation (and my sobriety) and put me in touch with others who in October of 2010 found me a consulting gig in Scranton, Pennsylvania. And as, "The Office" proclaimed, there's no party like a Scranton party. That's a joke if the sarcasm didn't translate. Scranton, PA is about as exciting as watching the polar ice caps melt. Holy hell is there nothing to do in Scranton. No wonder it's a former blue collar, drinking town, that almost everyone has vacated except the people born and raised there who don't have enough money to move away. Sorry, Scranton, I guess I won't be getting the key to your city. Turns out there were some positives weaved into my Scranton consulting gig. I lived, five days a week at the Hilton in downtown Scranton that was very nice. It was about 2 – 2.5 hours from Collegeville, so I'd drive up on a Sunday night and stayed until Friday (checking out Friday morning) and driving home to Collegeville after work. I was still morbidly obese BUT I was sober. While I was in Scranton I found several great AA meetings and when I came home to Collegeville on the weekends I went to meetings while I was at home to avoid the temptation to hang out continuously with my close friends at the bar, which is all they did, for the most part.

This consulting assignment only lasted about three months no thanks to the goofball who was running the project but whatever, it bridged a short term gap that I desperately needed at the time. I came home to Collegeville in January of 2010 and continued to go to meetings until February. February marked my six months in AA. Got my six-month coin and said to myself, "OK, I got this, I can drink responsibly, I am not an alcoholic I am simply a 'heavy drinker' as they speak about in the program." So, in February, I fell off the wagon and slowly began to drink again. After not drinking for six months, I can tell you that it didn't take much to get me hammered; so this also made me feel like I could control the situation because I wasn't able to drink more than two or three drinks without being shit faced. Seemed like a good control mechanism. Hell, I was even getting interviews for full-time positions at the time, so it must be OK with the karma Gods that I'm drinking again. Surely they would punish me if I was doing something wrong. Karma's only a bitch if you are! I heard that recently and I'm going to use it for a long time to come.

I interviewed for and obtained a full-time job in Basking Ridge, New Jersey in April of 2010. The position required me to be living in New Jersey so after 17 years in the Collegeville, Pennsylvania area it was time for me to move on. I moved to Hillsborough, New Jersey and moved into a similar apartment to what I had in Collegeville at the time. My girlfriend and I (who was living in Wilmington, Delaware at the time) tried our best to stay together but being an hour apart (PA to DE) was difficult. Being 2.5 hours away from north NJ to DE was damn near impossible. After a few months in NJ I had to be honest with her and with myself. I couldn't keep up the travel and I truly felt that I needed to spend time on Dale. This was the beginning of my epiphany that

I described earlier. It's now coming up on the June timeframe of 2010. At this point, refer back to the story of how 2010 (prior to my epiphany) unfolded. In case it wasn't already painfully obvious, my drinking since moving to New Jersey did not abate. It ramped up after my girlfriend and I split up. That's OK, it was leading up to my argument with my doctor in November. It allowed me to once again, at the beginning of my healthy journey, to determine that it was once again time to enter the program in January of 2011 directly after returning from Key West and coinciding with my nutrionalist and personal trainer. I knew going into "the program" this time; however, that I was fairly certain (although not completely convinced) that I'm still not an alcoholic; but my doctor was unfortunately right that I was a "heavy drinker" and a "binge drinker." I knew, with the help of the program and the amazing people that are a part of the whole AA culture, experience, group, and family that I would not be alone and that I had people to lean on. I went into the groups with a firm commitment of not picking up a drink until my birthday in June (five months). While in the program I waffled as to whether or not I could continue it beyond June. I truly wanted to but the progress I made in my first five months of personal training and diet modification were so amazing that when I hit my 42nd birthday, I celebrated by going to a new nudist resort I had never been to in the eastern mountains of West Virginia and ended up having my first glass of wine. Thankfully, by the point, my dietician had made me such a calorie Nazi that it was easy to not over-drink. Quick aside: If you're Jewish and take offense to my use of the word Nazi in reference to my calorie counting than I suggest you use that anger to do some cardio and stop stuffing matzo balls down your gullet. If you haven't picked up on my brutal honestly and my sense of humor by now, than for God's sake get over yourself. I couldn't afford the calories.

Since June of 2011, moderation is not just the name of the game for me; it's all about the calories and continues to be, to this day. What my friends from AA and other anonymous groups will appreciate is that being a calorie Nazi on alcohol enabled me to make one decision that I have never regretted. When I returned to having alcohol in June of 2011, I vowed to myself I would only ever consume wine or VERY light beer. My initial pledge was "wine weekends only" and I've almost entirely stuck with that philosophy since then. Since June of 2011, I can count on one hand the number of beers I've had that are not Michelob Ultras (95 calories, 2.5g of carbs). I have not, since January 2, 2011, ever again touched a drop of any hard liquor from whiskey to vodka. This was difficult but the calories made it a no-brainer and time has made it a habit. I have tried other programs with a 12-step approach as well and I've found some of them helpful. If you think you're eating habits or unhealthy issues may relate to a dysfunctional upbringing, you may want to check out Adult Children of Alcoholics (ACoA or ACA = same thing – don't tell them I said that). Your parents didn't necessarily have to be alcoholics although there may have been other dysfunctions in the home ranging from drugs to other physical or psychological (emotional) abuse. SLAA (or simply SexAA or LoveAA) is another one I've dipped my toe in and while I think it's a fantastic program, it has such a negative stereotype that it's difficult to share strength and hope outside of the circle of those involved. Depending on the area you live (such as mine) the choice of meetings is slim. I found ACA a great compromise while sharing some of the same principals of other 12-step programs; but it focuses on living your life for you, not others. Just telling you what worked for me, you don't have to accept or even pay attention to this piece of advice.

So, when I returned from Key West with a few things spinning through my head, I could no longer fight the wave that was coming over me. "Bitch Tits," "Cardio, cardio, cardio," a total of a year in AA, and the 12 steps are ringing me with "you can't do this alone," "use half the money you'd spend on me on a personal trainer." January 6, 2011 (five days after my return from Key West and five days into my second stint at total sobriety), I put down $600 for 20 one-hour training sessions with Chris Gaffney (lawyers probably have to get this release, too) who was the male personal trainer at the gym I belonged to at the time. January 14, 2011 I also started seeing Mary Ellen McCrea, RD in Somerville, NJ. Huge reveal for the book… Without the help/ encouragement/push of Chris, Mary Ellen, Kevin (more on Kevin later), Dr. Glatt's lack of help (a good thing), Dr. T (my regular doctor who I argued about my alcohol problem), none of this would have been possible. As Chris was always so good at reminding me… "…you're the one doing it Dale; no one else is doing it." Yes, he was spot-on, but when you are climbing a mountain or driving a car in a race, there's a group of people supporting you that are keys to your success and without them you'd be nothing/nowhere.

PT

Shortly after signing on my personal trainer, Chris, I knew I needed help with "the other 50 percent." My firm and fundamental belief is that the trick to significant weight loss is a 50/50 effort between diet and exercise. There are many secrets to unlock on both sides of the equation. Most people think the food/diet is more complicated than the exercise, but this is not the case. They are equally difficult because while you think you know how to work out, you don't. While you think you "might be able to motivate yourself," you can't. And no matter how good of a high school or collegiate athlete you were you aren't any more. Running is a science. This isn't Nike in 1972. You don't melt some rubber on your wife's waffle iron strap them to your feet with some leather laces and just go running like the Kenyan you saw at the last Olympics. It's a bit more technical than that. Running is composed of cadence, posture, foot pronation/supination, compression gear, lack of cotton (clothing), technique, base building, speed training, heart rate levels, incline/decline approach/attack, hydration, glucose intake, VO_2 max, proper footwear and other areas and this is just running. We haven't gotten into biking, swimming, elliptical, stair climbing, cross fit, Zumba, or any other cardio fit exercise. Diet is just as complicated and it can be just as oversimplified as exercise. Eat less! Goes back to my simple formula; "more out than in." Duh! No shit Sherlock! If it was that simple 80 percent of America wouldn't be FAT!

Dietician

So let's talk about a dietician versus a nutrionalist. When I retained the services of a professional I admit that it had a lot to do with who my health plan referred me to; but while I got REAL lucky with Mary Ellen (who is a Registered Dietician – RD), I will not throw a nutrionalist under the bus either. However, the fact of the matter is that a nutrionalist isn't a legal term and technically just because someone says they are a nutrionalist, it doesn't mean they're educated or qualified to provide you advice to assist you in living a healthy lifestyle. With that said, if someone is "hanging their shingle" out with the claim they are a nutrionalist and someone goes to see them for advice, they are staking their own reputation, business, and potentially livelihood on their recommendations. A registered dietician is usually a person who is in someone affiliated with a hospital, health plan, or other health related organization.

According to the Academy of Nutrition and Dietetics (United States), a registered dietician is someone who has:

- Earned a bachelor's degree with course work approved by the Academy of Nutrition and Dietetics' Accreditation Council for Education in Nutrition and Dietetics.
- Completed an accredited, supervised practice program at a healthcare facility, community agency or foodservice corporation.
- Passed a national examination administered by the Commission on Dietetic Registration.
- Completed continuing professional educational requirements to maintain registration.

A registered dietitian may plan food and nutrition programs and promote healthy-eating habits to prevent and treat illness. They often work in food service or as part of medical teams in hospitals, clinics and other healthcare facilities. Dietitians also work in university settings, where they may teach, do research or focus on public health issues.

A nutritionist is someone who's studied nutrition and may have a graduate degree (M.S. or Ph.D.) in nutrition from an accredited college. Dietitians are considered to be nutritionists, but not all nutritionists are dietitians. Some healthcare providers (medical doctors, osteopaths, physician assistants, chiropractors and naturopathic doctors) may be considered to be nutritionists if they've completed extra study in the area of nutrition and they may practice "clinical nutrition." This type of nutrition is often considered part of alternative or complementary medicine. While only a dietitian can use the title "dietician," it's important to understand that the term "nutritionist" itself is not protected, so, in regions where nutrition and dietetics are not licensed or regulated, anyone can call themselves a nutritionist, even if they're not qualified.

The first thing Mary Ellen had me do was "not change anything" for two weeks. Just document every single piece of ANYTHING that went into my fat mouth. The only thing she didn't care about was water. Well, that was easy as I didn't drink much of that. Actually, I was drinking "fizzy" like it was "going out of style." That is, flavored seltzer water. I had given up alcohol (at least for the short-term) by this point, but my 3,000 calorie per day diet was horrible and she knew it; but I needed to understand the magnitude of it. We considered the alcohol I had just given up when we were figuring out the 3,000 per day number. After two weeks of documenting everything from sauces to meats, cheeses, crappy fried food, fast food, etc... we sat down and started to put calories on my daily food log that I had been filling out. When she initially said we were going to cut my intake to 1,500 – 1,800 calories a day I had no concept of what that meant. OK, with alcohol I was at 3,000 calories per day and without it I was probably at 2500 +/-. Yes, geniuses, go figure out how much 500 calories of alcohol is per day and many of you will say that wasn't bad, except I didn't drink much during the week. Maybe a beer a night plus my "night, night juice" was usually a double to triple shot of Jameson Irish Whiskey. GODDAMN IT, I loved my Jameson. We were asshole buddies, Jameson and I. What a messy ugly divorce that was.

Mary Ellen took complete advantage of my profession (I mentioned I'm a computer geek – well, I'm a manager of IT geeks these days but I'm still a geek at heart). She knew if she could tap into my OCD, anal retentive, spreadsheet master I would be hooked. DAMN her, she was so right. I hope she gives me permission to publish her name in this book and reads this section. That god damn food log she had me start filling out on January 14, 2011 has turned into (as of this writing) over 150 separate Excel spreadsheets (one per week) since then. Correct, pick ANY day in the last three years and I can tell you EXACTLY what I had to eat on that day and how many calories I consumed. Overkill, yes. Unnecessary at this point, yes. OCD? Anal retentive? Yes. A part of the way I "choose" to manage my life, yes. And it's a positive one for a change. I don't beat myself up anymore if I'm a little off but I am still just as religious about planning my weekly meals. More about that in a little bit.

I need to address a few fundamentals from my year with Mary Ellen. KISS = Keep it simple, stupid. Convenient, as this is a philosophy of my own personal life as well. This is what we did. It's going to take time and your body is going to figure it out. Her statement, "I don't care if you do drink 1,500 calories in alcohol per day but once you hit 1,500 calories for the day, you're done. PERIOD! Now go! Your body will figure it out. Come see me in two weeks and I'll give you some suggestions." Realistically, she gave me some suggestions out of the chute, but every time I'd go back (every two weeks) she'd offer additional suggestions to continually drive me in the right direction. She was as much a therapeutical counselor as she was a dietician. Let me describe KISS. You've probably heard the acronym before, but let me translate it into nutritional speak. I will preface this with my usual legal disclaimer. I had no medical issues or prescription drugs other than some food allergies that I knew to avoid. If you have any medical conditions that you are seeing a doctor or are on medication, you need to consult them before taking my word as gospel but (huge but) my words are also not going to be far off from what your doctor will otherwise tell you. Remember the title of the book, "Everything your mother told you…" For 99.999 percent of the audience reading this book, you're mom was not a rocket scientist, so even she knew the right thing to do. So, KISS… 1,500 – 1,800 calories per day was challenging enough for a guy who didn't know there was a label with serving sizes on the back on almost every single thing you can put in your body.

Do I have to look at fats, carbs, proteins, sugars, minerals, cholesterol, sodium, and other categories? No, KISS, all we care about is calories. All those other indicators are important, don't get me wrong. They will have a much larger impact if you ignore them, but if you're where I was (and you probably are – i.e. FAT) and you're trying to lose weight and you're following my calorie and exercise plan than the "other factors" will sort themselves out. So, this is what I did from January 2011 until I lost my goal weight by November of 2011. Nine months saw about a 75 – 80 pound reduction. I wasn't done losing weight, but I far exceeded any and all of the goals I had set for myself with Mary Ellen and Chris's help. From 235 pounds my first goal was to simply be under 200. That would be a small miracle. When I hit 199 I cried but I knew I could hit 195. When I hit 195 I said it was going to be hard but I could reach the top end of my BMI at 185. OMG, what would that look like? I'd be 55 pounds less than when I started. I'd be at a "normal" BMI for the first time in probably 20 years. When I surpassed 185 on my way to 175, Mary Ellen tried to slow me up saying I was losing a little too much too fast and she was worried I wouldn't be able to maintain it and I could have severe negative consequences.

I slowed down and maintained a weight in the 170s for a month, but I REALLY wanted to get to the low end of my BMI at 165. I knew it was within reach and I knew I could get there I just had to convince Mary Ellen that I could do it, maintain it and still be happy with my success. So 165 = 70 pounds lost over about eight months. I fantasized during this time… Could I actually see the 150s? I knew Mary Ellen was actually against me going below my BMI, but I also think she may have under-estimated my newly found freedom and love of being an athlete. I hit 159 and I remember her not being happy. At this point, after 8.5 months it was a game to me. I was so in control of my body and my intake/output that I could control a few pounds at will over the period of a week or two. I added a couple pounds back on so she wouldn't be too upset that I was getting "too skinny." I'm not anorexic but I know she had patients/clients with that issue, so I was sensitive to where she was coming from. It was around this time (about eight months into seeing her) where we scaled down to monthly visits and I said, why don't I "call you if I need some advice" but I think I got it from here. Wow, did I have it. I was free to experiment and play with the numbers. So, I did. I "bottomed out" at 155 pounds. That's 80 pounds lost over a period of about 9.5 months. This was below my BMI but into the "athletic" category. I gave myself an opportunity to make sure I could sustain it and that I wasn't just doing it to look skinny. Mary Ellen was always big on making sure your body "feels right." No one's body feels right FAT but if your ideal BMI is between 165 and 185 pounds than you may feel comfortable and OK, anywhere in that range depending on your overall fitness and activity level. OK, well, I felt comfortable at 155. I have since dipped, at most, to 149 but never below. I maintain my weight (2.5 years later) between 150 – 158 pounds depending on races I may be entered into on any given dates. The longer the race I'm entering the higher the number. The shorter the race I'm running the lower I like to be to the bottom of this range.

I've talked about the argument with my doctor and going into AA for the first five months of my kick start to this new healthy lifestyle. I've also mentioned that as a computer guy for a living, I'm fairly numbers oriented and a logical person by nature. The reason I reiterate this here is that I believe that a part of every person's plan to get healthy should include this fundamental approach to achieve your goals. That is, if you are going to do something for yourself that you alone were not able to handle in the past but with the help of this book, a Higher Power, and your own personal desire to stop the vicious cycle of self-abuse, you need to be honest and **identify your demons**. Every single person reading this book has demons. Whether you are fat, obese or know someone who is obese, you have your demons. These demons are the "bad angels," "dark spot on our brain," the "black hat," or the evil subconscious. These demons are what enable, foster, sustain, create havoc, provoke, incite, engage, control (oh, that's a big one – control), or lose control over our healthy choices, positive or negative.

My demon, as you've probably already figured out, was alcohol. I do not deny that I had a problem with alcohol. I make no excuses for it. I may have had some negative influences along the way (oh boy did I), but I am still responsible for my own actions and decisions. I had negative influences from the time I was 13 (probably before but I don't remember much before 13) until the age of 41 when I moved to New Jersey. That's a long time to punish oneself (28 years of self-abuse through unhealthy lifestyle choices). OK, back to demons. Here's the simple, unabridged, in your face style of my book. I don't give a shit what your demons are. It doesn't matter. Anyone else (other than me) on this planet may think they're the dumbest, weirdest, most mentally disturbed thing they've ever heard, <u>but if it's your demon and it prohibits you from making healthy lifestyle choices than you need to cut it out of your life, cold turkey, for six months</u>. Your internal computer/ hard drive is corrupted with an un-repairable virus. You need to reboot/ reimage the system. You need to wipe the hard drive clean (format it) and return to an original state of well-being. So, what's your demon? Let me throw out a shopping list of potential demons. Alcohol, cheese, chocolate, bread, fried food, fast food, red meat, pork, salt, your wife's nagging, your husband's laziness, your parents treatment of you like a child, your lack of self-esteem, pasta, ice cream, workaholic, smoking, drugs, gambling, sex, abandonment, porn, gaming, butter, sauces, oil, processed food, TV dinners, fear of sweat, fear of smelling bad, intimidation by others (or self) of "working out," pride, cookies, cupcakes, desserts, weather, or maybe it's just alcohol. I'm positive I missed about 1,000 demons, but I'm hopeful you got the point. It's not just food that are our demons, although I honestly find that this is almost at least in the top two things that hold people back from a truly healthy lifestyle. You're thinking that sure, I would potentially murder another human being for the perfect piece of chocolate cake, but I'm not addicted. It's not like I need to go to a Chocoholic Anonymous meeting. However, if you sit and meditate for a brief time you will land on your demon. Maybe it is chocolate and maybe it's not an addiction, but does is disable all the other mechanisms in your head that tell you it's OK to be healthy. Is the consumption of chocolate or the thought of a smelly gym/ locker room enough to motivate you, even inspire you, to avoid healthy decisions and even make potentially harmful decisions as a justification of your sickness? You can overcome any demon.

I feel a necessary disclaimer coming on as some of the mental issues I avoided in my shopping list above included things like depression, suicidal thoughts, self-mutilation, any other mental disorder more commonly treated with medication, or any physiological ailment treated by a physician. For instance, if you said your demon was diabetes; I would not accept that as your demon. Go back to my chapter on excuses. Diabetes is an excuse. You can control diabetes. You can control (with medication and a physician) almost any of your psychological or physiological issues. These are not your demons. If you got diabetes because you eat sugar like most people breathe air than you need to define your demon as sugar and your diabetes as an excuse. If you genetically inherited your diabetes than it's still an excuse you're using. Probe deeper, you'll find your demon. Find out what inhibits a healthy lifestyle. It may not come right away but if you meditate on it and start using some of my suggestions for healthy living you will discover your demon and then you can go back and kick its ass.

Again, rid yourself of this demon/system virus. Reboot your body. Six months without this demon will give you a new- found respect for yourself and your ability to slay this dragon. In the meantime, you'll be eating better, getting more exercise, losing weight, and gaining a whole new you (mentally and physically). If you can't do it alone I guarantee there's a support group out there somewhere that can help you. They have them for everything so if dressing up as a stuffed animal and having sex with the costume on is your demon that prevents you from a healthy lifestyle then, guess what? There's a plushophiles support group out there to help you (avoid the behavior not engage in it). If it was food, in six months, it won't taste the same and with any luck it'll either not taste good to you any more or you'll have realized that you have power over it, not the other way around. Similar to some of the mental issues I've learned to deal with in my own recovery, we often have to realize that we're surrendering control to the thing that's hurting us. The question is not, "why is this person or thing controlling me when I don't want them/it to?" A better question is most likely, "why am allowing this person or thing to have control over me?" Why am I "relinquishing control" to this thing? It doesn't deserve to control me. If I am giving control to another person who probably has their own demons, I may need to seriously look at that relationship. While I'm not suggesting you eliminate another person from your life for six months, I am saying that if you mentioned another person as your demon you may need to explain to that person that you're going to spend the next months focused on yourself; and this may cause some stress on the relationship, but if you do not do it they may not have you much longer anyway.

Let me discuss a few things about my diet before, during, and after my transition to healthy living and where I stand today on my journey. I know I'm not at the end of this journey of learning yet, but I know many things will take time to accept and adjust to. As of this writing I've been following a progressively healthier diet for three years. It took me the first 18 months (1.5 years) to finally put an end to red meat in my diet. I don't do it because I care about the animals, the cruelty to the animal, the cholesterol (although that's something to consider), or the 50 other reasons people give for avoiding red meat. Remember, KISS. There's an average of 60 calories per ounce or red meat versus 27 calories per ounce for chicken. It's easy peezy lemon squeezy. I can have twice as much chicken as steak. Simple, not complicated. After 18 months, I finally embodied the quote that fewer legs are always better. If your meat source has four legs, it's not as healthy as an animal that only has two legs, and if the animal has no legs (fish) it's the best. No, I'm not talking about cutting the legs off cows and chickens to make them healthier you silly goose. Would I someday like to even move away from chicken/turkey as my mainstay protein source? Sure, I'd like to think I'm working towards it by incorporating more quinoa and lentils in my weekly diet as much better sources of protein than meat. With that said, making fish for lunch a few days in advance and re-heating it for lunch every day is like having your family stay over for a week vacation. It's OK for a few days, but starts to stink by day four (literally).

I will show some examples of my weekly diet from various stages of my "growth" in healthy living. I will include the Microsoft Excel template as either a part of this book or upon request to my web site (I sure hope someone can redo mine by the time I get this book published www.dalebondanza.com). I've probably stated it at least once or twice that your transition to healthy living must be gradual. Like so many other life lessons, if you rush it you will not succeed in the long- term. You may lose some weight but you will not keep it off. You may be able to run a 5K but you may get injured, depressed or rest on your laurels. Healthy living is a journey not a destination. How freaking hack is that statement? But, it's true nonetheless. Off the top of my head I want to quote some of the diet stages I went through on my journey to date. When Mary Ellen initially set my goal as 1,500 – 1,800 calories for the day it was damned difficult to figure out how I wasn't going to starve with that much of a reduction in daily intake. Of course, the alcohol reduction was huge but still not nearly enough. Even if alcohol accounted for 500 – 600 calories a day (that was an average – it really wasn't that much during the week) then I still had to find 700 +/- calories to cut from other places. My initial lessons mainly revolved around learning calories in everything I picked up. I read EVERY label (get used to it and you'll always do it). You don't have to over focus on every nutritional element of the food. Just look at calories. Compare two items that you want to eat and take the lesser calories. This was my first lesson. My second lesson and more important in the long run was the bane of every red-blooded American: **portion size/control.**

The average order for Chinese takeout should be enough to last you four meals. Can you think of the last time you saved it for more than one? Maybe you even saved it for a lunch and dinner the following day. That's great. More often than not you sat down in front of the TV with your take out and ate the whole thing like a dog. It's OK, you're American. How many fat Chinese people do you see? That's what you say in your fat head. Do you ever consider that's not what they eat, just what they're trying to kill us with so they can take over the planet? And you're letting them, you idiot. I bet many of you love Chinese but wouldn't consider Japanese sushi something any American should eat. Guess what, so did "fat Dale." I'd have eaten horse asshole before sushi. Two and half years later I can finally not only enjoy sushi but occasionally try sashimi. Quick education… Sushi is not raw it's actually cooked seafood (when there's even seafood in it). Sashimi is truly raw fish. There are a ton of sushi rolls that have no fish in them at all. Some have crab, lobster or shrimp that even you fatties like. Who doesn't like lobster or shrimp dripping in butter? Now wrap that yummy up with some rice and a couple vegetables to make it look healthy/appetizing and charge $8 for it. Bingo! But I digress.

Back to portion control. *Read the goddamn label.* Did I say that already? Did I tell you to buy a food scale? You're going to want one eventually – doesn't need to be fancy, but get something (preferably digital) that tells you weight in grams and ounces. This is so handy and necessary to healthy living. You need to grow a respect for two ounces of pasta. It's an OK food (as carbs go) but you must respect the portion. It's true for corn and or peas, too. You eat corn on the cob or regular corn out of a can and think because you're eating a vegetable you're doing something healthy. Corn, for me, went the way of red meat. Crazy I know, but don't worry; you'll enjoy it again someday when you learn to control your fatness. Meat should never exceed the size of your fist. Your fist is approximately six ounces unless you have meat hooks (no pun intended). If you do, use the scale to figure out what six ounces is. You can have six ounces of protein (meat) with each main meal (lunch / dinner). What about breakfast you ask? It reminds me of one of my favorite quotes from the Simpsons that I'll purposely get wrong so they won't sue me. From Homer to Lisa, "Sure Lisa, bacon, pork chops, sausage, ham, and pork ribs all come from the same mystical animal, sure they do." To which Lisa's response is, "DAD!!!"

Another very valuable lesson I learned on my journey, especially for the first 9+ months, was that just because it's lower in calories doesn't mean it's "good for you." Remember my mission, get skinny and to reduce total calories, come hell or high water. Well, I did and I did that with whatever products I could eat and still enjoy the taste of without feeling too much like I was on a diet. This came through my new found love of Thai food and all things sausage. After all, how bad can something called "Al Fresca Chicken Sausage" be for your diet? First of all, it was way tastier than I imagined possible. And, the calories were WAY lower than I had been eating with all the red meat. Since I was into all things sausage I allowed myself to have Italian sausage at least once per week as well. I limited the portion as I had learned, but still allowed myself to have it. Both my dietician and personal trainer hinted that maybe I should start to look beyond simple calories, but they also didn't completely object because they knew I was focused on the calories; and since I was exercising as much as I was (five days a week at this point) they could let the other unhealthy aspects of sausage slide (for now).

There are a couple of "stages" I need to talk about that every person will encounter on their journey to healthy living. You will go through stages of food that are progressively healthier. You will be eating one type of food for months thinking this is awesome that you're being so healthy, and eventually you'll grow tired of eating the same thing or realize there are "side effects" that don't always outweigh the benefits. This should be apparent from my last paragraph about chicken sausage or my absolute favorite for six months (turkey kielbasa). OMG! I thought turkey kielbasa was manna from heaven. Low calories, turkey, and damn tasty – what could be bad? Eventually, I gave in and looked at those other silly lines on the label like sodium and well, sodium. What the hell did I need to look at (from the beginning) but refused to get past the calories and the fact that I could have 3.5 servings and it was still allowable as a protein source for one meal. PERFECT! And, why should I care, my blood pressure from all the working out obviously wasn't affected by the amount of sodium in this product. Or, was it? Once I realized that my once per week serving of turkey kielbasa gave me 2000 percent of my daily sodium intake I decided that this manna should "probably" be replaced by turkey burgers. Eventually, the same thing happened with the chicken sausage, which became skinless, boneless, chicken breast with just the proper amount of zero calorie dry rub seasoning. As you were reading the previous paragraph you were probably screaming at me and to yourself. He's eating processed food, how can that be good for you? No shit Sherlock! I know that now, and may have even known it at the time, but the point of my whole book is that this is a journey of continuous learning. It takes time. If the above process is how I slowly reduced my calories and got away from red meat and someday leads me away from all meat, than that was the right journey for me. Maybe you can learn from my mistakes. Maybe you should be as lucky to make the same mistakes. Maybe you'll make exactly the same mistakes. If it gets you to healthy, it doesn't matter how you get there, just get there.

I can even talk about the obviously healthy things I did that were still fads (to be repeated again someday as they're very healthy and positive); but as I said earlier, sometimes you get sick of the same ol' shit day in and day out. Reminds me of a few of my girlfriends... HA, just kidding dears (not really but they knew who they were). Green grapes, apples, and bananas have been staples for the longest time. My daily snack was green grapes for the better part of the first year. I would buy them in bulk, de-stem them and freeze half while the others became my nightly "snack food" to keep my calories up when I needed to raise my calories for the day. An apple and banana were in my lunch EVERY day for almost the first 1.5 years of my diet. I bought two apple coring tools (one for work and one for home) that I used to cut my Granny Smith apples EVERY day. It was the same with the bananas. I'm not going to say I can never look at a Granny Smith or banana again. I quite like them both, but every day got tiring. For many months now I have opted to buy the pre-cut up fruit sold at my local grocery store and dish eight ounces of that out every day (100 calories) with a 140 cup of Greek yogurt. It's the perfect combination of protein and fruit and an awesome 240 calories snack or dessert to a main meal.

Here's the perfect example of something that went by the wayside and has now made it back into my cupboard even as I sit here and type this paragraph. It's quite humorous actually. Back when I couldn't get enough calories in my daily routine because I needed 2,700 per day, I was often searching for my nightly snacks. A healthy suggestion from my dietician (Mary Ellen) was Apple Cinnamon Cheerios. Three quarters of a cup for 120 calories. It's a great snack with no need for milk or anything else to mess it up. Just eat it dry like a snack and it's yummy.

Let's talk about some other phases, treats, and cooking phases I went through. Here are a couple of easy ones that will allow you fatties to breathe a little sign of relief. Guess what, if you work hard, you will be rewarded (sounds like something your mother would say, right)? Well, it's true for following my path as well. When I began this transformation process in Hillsborough, I found a local restaurant next to my local grocery store that would become a staple of rewarding myself that holds true to this day. After I lost the bulk of the weight, I started to make it my EVERY Saturday dinner. It was a delicious little Thai restaurant. I didn't even know I liked Thai food until I tried this place. OMG! Let me mention a huge side note here. For years, as a fat guy, I had the worse Irritable Bowel Syndrome (IBT). Realistically, my body wasn't processing the crap I was putting into it and it was rebelling on me by taking otherwise delicious (especially tasty food) and throwing it out of my asshole with a path of destruction in its wake. You weren't eating while you were reading that were you? Now that I'm healthy, SURPRISE, spicy food and the occasional "bad food" doesn't bother me like it did because my body may not like it, but it doesn't rebel against it now either. It says, "I have no idea why you just had a small order of French fries, but I'll take the usable calories and deposit the rest in your colon fairly quickly." While Thai food is still a huge reward for being a good boy it is not my every Saturday meal anymore. I have learned (especially now that I live in Florida) that grilling fish (Chilean sea bass, mahi mahi, lobster, shrimp, etc…) is an even better/ healthier route for me to go. Another note that I learned within the scope of my weekly Thai reward was the most awesome rice I've EVER tasted. The Thai use primarily white jasmine rice. This has become my carb staple. One half cup of jasmine rice for my lunch and dinner meals (about 160 – 180 calories) is the perfect starch. I don't have it every day or every week, but I've learned to use it because it's easy and quick to prepare and can be used as a double starch on the days leading up to a race.

Cooking phases is an interesting subject. Here's the order the two-year self-cooking journey took. There was the Mini Grill, Small George Foreman, Large George Forman, Mini Grill, Large George Forman (move to Florida)… so grill, grill, grill, grill. OK, this was only true for all of my proteins (meats). Even during my phases of "healthy chicken sausage" grilling on the George Forman did make sense because it took much of the fat that was in these foods and got rid of them naturally. What about all the other food fads. Well, to be honest a fad that isn't a fad is microwavable steamed vegetables. These are a godsend to the healthy eater. Another fad that branched out was the starch source. Literally, for over the first year the jasmine rice I mentioned above was a daily staple of my diet. I had a half cup or rice two times per day Monday through Friday. I bought a 40-pound bag of rice at the local grocery store. Forty pounds of rice makes 80 pounds. This much rice lasted me more than four months of having it "almost" every day. Many days I used a "wrap" as my starch just to change it up a little. I'd use the wrap to make a quasi-sandwich out of my turkey burger, tofu, or chicken breast.

One more food phase that I want to describe because it's going to sound a little crazy to some… OK, maybe it isn't crazy to think that someone who's getting healthy would enjoy salads a few times a week instead of their regular protein, starch, and vegetable meal. I would say, that for the first 22 months of my diet plan I used almost every Monday and Tuesday lunch meal as my salad meal. Why was it a phase? Because I stopped doing it after that time because I had finally figured out that my body was not doing well with the amount of roughage I was putting into it; that is, it needed more solid foods because I was exercising so much and running so far that leafy things processed way too fast through my system. Spinach leaves in particular. Spinach was processed so quickly through my system I finally just started throwing it into the toilet to avoid the "middle man." Seemed like less hassle. Kidding, of course, but I have not missed my salad phase. Let me talk more about why it was and is a necessary evil to help you train and reboot your body away from the fats of your daily living. EVERYONE knows that salads are good for you. However, when you go to a salad bar, or you see a fat cow eating a salad, you look at them and instantly say, "Well, at least (s)he's trying." Do you ever take a second look to see that the poor salad is being covered, completely, choked out, by the cheese, dressing, croutons, buffalo chicken, and assorted other various things that just took this 250 calorie salad and made it an 800 calorie disaster in hiding. No, it's not a nice try. It's called fooling yourself and you need to be called out on this shit behavior. Almost allowable if you excluded the cheese and croutons and went with oil and balsamic vinegar instead of the dressing.

Even if you do the O&V option remember that a good EVOO (Extra Virgin Olive Oil) is still 99 calories per tablespoon. The balsamic is usually around 34 calories per tablespoon so two tablespoons of vinegar and one tablespoon of EVOO is enough for four cups of salad. Did I say four cups? Holy lettuce Batman that's a lot of salad you're saying. Yes you fat pig, it is. It's also only about 30 calories. Go for the bulk of that much salad and you won't need all the other crap you're piling on the damn thing to make you "think" you're being healthy. For my 22 months of salad fetish I always put six ounces of protein on the salad. Either steak or chicken was my typical protein. I typically put steak on it for the first year of my diet and then moved to steak on one day and chicken on the other. After 18 months went to chicken on both days until I eliminated the salad all together. Don't be confused. Here was my typical Monday/Tuesday lunch salad. Four cups of salad (the mixed stuff that comes in a bad at the grocery store) contains about 10 calories per serving with four servings in a bag. Have the whole bag. I know, it's a lot. No, it's only about 40 calories. One slice of low fat cheddar cheese singles (25 calories). Six ounces of protein (let's say steak to make it bulk up) equals 360 calories. One whole bell pepper chopped (31 calories) sounds like a lot but again, you're going for bulk here. Oil and Vinegar (one tablespoon/two tablespoons) respectively is 99 plus 68 calories. This is a good Monday salad.

On Tuesday I would use chicken (162 calories instead of the 360) and mushrooms (eight ounces) instead of the whole pepper that is actually less (about 15 calories). So, therefore, total calorie count for Monday salad was: 40 + 25 +360 + 31 +99 + 68 = 623 calories of a perfectly balanced salad. Admittedly, Tuesday's salad was much healthier but I needed time to adjust and the steak on Monday let me slowly make that transition. Remember, it took me a YEAR to convert to chicken only. This is not simple. I know what it's like to love red meat. I was you for forty (40)+ years. I know what I'm asking of you. If I did it, so can you. Tuesday's salad was a slightly lower: 40 + 25 +162 + 15 +99 + 68 = 409 calories. You can't eat peppers? You're disgusted by raw mushrooms? Pick whatever "salad bar topping" you want as long as it doesn't exceed 31 or 15 calories. Hell, you can pick croutons or nuts or oranges but if you only get to have one crouton, one tablespoon of pine nuts, or 1/16 of an orange and you'll understand why bulk is better. BUT, if that's the way you have to go to ease yourself into it, than just don't go over those calorie numbers and your body will slowly adjust. You will find, as you lose weight and begin to like what you see in the mirror that you may develop a new taste for something (mushrooms) you previous thought was disgusting. Hmm, I can have eight ounces of mushrooms for the same "cost" as one crouton. Let me think about that, OK, thought about it, mushrooms aren't so bad.

Here's a fad that lasted less than one month, but it was all I needed to kick myself in the head hard enough to expand my knowledge of nutrition and bring myself to that "next level" or healthy living/eating. I've spoken about a ton of food fads I've had over my diet journey, but none was shorter or made more of an impression than the month that Kevin (he hasn't gotten much mention yet but will soon) convinced me to really examine the major components of what I was eating beyond just the basic calories and serving size. He convinced me to expand the scope of my spreadsheet analysis to include carbs, protein, fats, and sodium content. That's it. There's plenty more he could have charged me with, but he limited it to these as he obviously knew this is where most of my issues laid. If you are also a fat bastard in transition maybe these are the same areas that affect you.

Maybe you need your dietician to be your "Kevin". Maybe, like me, you just need to read the WHOLE label and stop trying to kid yourself that just because it's lower in calories doesn't mean it's good for you. There are degrees to healthy living. I was clearly at a point where I needed to take the next step, and Kevin wanted to kick my ass to that stage instead of waiting for me to discover it. Thank you Kevin! I'll take a slight pause to be emotional for a second. I was wasting precious time on my journey to healthy living and to think that I probably wasted about four to six months makes me sad, but I chalk it up to experience and the knowledge (albeit after the fact) that I knew I was wrong when I was doing it and should have trusted myself. Chicken sausage, Italian sausage, turkey kielbasa may have been lower in calories, but their sodium content was off the charts. I also wasn't getting the amount of protein I needed for the types of training/workouts Kevin was putting me through. They were all body weight resistance and functional exercises specific to running and building core. Carbs were carbs. I was learning, at this phase of my training, that carbs are not the enemy of a runner (or someone who does as much cardio as I was doing).

Refined sugars (fats) are the enemy. Focus on the proper amount of carbs and protein while minimizing the fats and sodium and your heart will thank you, your core will thank you and your body, overall, will thank you. Hell, your asshole may even begin to forgive years of putting up with your IBT because you thought McDonald's French fries and $1 cheeseburgers were the cure to hangovers (well, they are but not for the right reasons). Anyway, this is a necessary phase of your transitional diet from fat, disgusting human to refined, healthy machine. You will go through it but I hope I've made you aware that when it comes time to analyze these factors, you speak with your dietician or nutritional coach about limiting sodium content in everything to less than 10 percent per serving. Make sure you have the right number of grams of protein and carbs based on your current weight for the amount of exercising you are doing. The formula is too complex to list in this book and I would violate my scientific basis for getting you healthy if I went into it. That is, you don't need to know anything more than you can Google on the subject. Google, "proper amount of carbs (or protein) for a XX year old (fe)male," and you will get some great reference calculators that you can use to figure these amounts out. Now, analyze your daily food intake for these proteins and carbs (and fats/sodium) to see where you can hone in on what you need to propel yourself to the next level.

Ode to KK

Here's my dedication to Kevin. I'm sitting here typing and even having four ounces of wine to loosen up my mind a little for writing; and when I started this paragraph I paused for a moment to reflect on my 6-plus month relationship with Kevin. I took a sip of wine, put my folded hands in my lap and stared at my forearms for a minute. I realize, as I'm staring at my arms that they would not look like this today if it wasn't for the work that Kevin (and Chris before him) put into me as a project. I can see every vein in both of my arms, and hands. This is how I know my protein and carb ratios are perfect. This is how I know my heart is continuously getting stronger. I said, as I was sitting here typing this, I should go check my blood pressure and pulse because I'm feeling really good and thankful right now. Good choice on my part. My blood pressure as I'm sitting here typing is 113/53 and my pulse rate is 53. That pulse rate is literally 50 percent of what it was two years ago. For your heart to beat less than one time every second means you have trained it for some intense action.

I love where I am today on my healthy journey. I have my current life and look and self-image thanks to Kevin (and Chris and Mary Ellen). You three are amazing and blessed for the gifts you've given so many, but I thank you from the bottom of my "runner's heart." Kevin wasn't even getting paid to help me. While I was working out in Hillsborough, Chris was my personal trainer at the gym, working for the club. He was getting paid by the club, but I was paying them for his time. Kevin was just one of the guys who worked behind the desk, but he was also an amazing, nationally ranked Iron Man who was fundamentally interested in helping me learn and enjoy running and simultaneously get sober (in every way possible). He took a personal interest. When Chris made the decision (so wise on his part) to leave NJ and move to South Florida I cried (literally), but wished him the best and hoped to soon follow. Kevin stepped up to the plate, became the new personal trainer at the gym and took over my case/cause. Chris was my undergraduate degree in getting healthy. Kevin certainly took me to the next level (master's degree) based on where Chris left off. Kevin befriended me outside the walls of the gym and without that friendship I would not be the man/runner I am today. Kevin is a blessed soul and I say that as a devout agnostic. Thank you, friend! Blessed be and peace. Without you (and Chris and Mary Ellen) there would be no "skinny Dale." Maybe this should be the foreword to my book but again, it seemed appropriate here. ☺

OK, so now, when I return I'd like to pre-address my diet worksheets. I've explained my plan. <u>It's a simple formula: **More out then in.**</u> **Remember, your steps to great health include: diet, exercise, 12-step program as necessary, Higher Power as necessary, personal trainer, dietician/ nutrionalist. These are fundamentals.** Everything else I present is inconsequential if you don't get these basic points.

<u>**Simple formula = More out than in.**</u> That is, you have to burn more calories than you consume to lose weight. This is a simple formula. Ignore credit cards, banks, and loan sharks for a minute… Unless you are the federal government you cannot spend more than you make. It's a similar formula. One pound = 3,500 calories. If you want to lose one pound per week you must have a deficit of 3,500 calories per week. That is if you consume 2,000 calories a day times seven days that = 14,000 calories. I will assume you're maintaining your weight at this calorie level. If you want to lose one pound of weight you must burn 17,500 calories. Again, it's a VERY simple formula so far, right? Here's some magic for you. If you are really eating 2,000 calories a day (you're probably not because you're fat and reading this book, but let's just go with it for a second) and you are maintaining your current weight guess what that means? If you are not gaining OR losing weight you are MAINTAINING your weight with a 2,000 calorie per day diet doing whatever "exercise" you're doing now. PERFECT, good job! You only need to burn another 3,500 calories to lose the one pound. And 3,500 calories over the course of one week = 3500 / 7 = 500 calories per day. Can you either eat less and/or burn more to lose that one pound. Sure, "piece of cake" (not literally). You can burn 300 calories with 30 minutes of aerobic exercise per day and eliminate the other 200 calories from your food intake. Did that make sense? I didn't go too fast with the math, right? I'm not trying to be a prick, I'm

serious. If you workout at an aerobic pace for 50 minutes you don't have to eliminate any calories at all.

OK, here's where you're starting to have some questions. Dale, you're telling me I need to workout EVERY day for 50 minutes to burn 500 calories? Yes, is that so hard to believe you fat pig? That's REALLY NOT THAT MUCH of an investment in your health. OK, I'll make it easier. Math has a way of doing that for you. You better thank me for the math trick I'm about to show you. If you really believe what I'm about to show you is magic please immediately go buy another 10 copies of this book and fling them at the head of other fat people like you're the head coach of Rutger's Basketball team. Here's the magic… If you're reading this book and you're as fat as I think you probably are you are NOT eating only 2,000 calories a day. You are probably closer to 2,600 or 3,000 or more. Let's say, just for giggles, that you still only want to lose one pound per week, therefore the same 3,500 calories per week or 500 calorie per day lose is required. Like magic now you only have to work out for 25 minutes per day as long as you eliminate 250 calories from your massive diet.

Don't tell anyone but here's the magic… 250 less calories + 25 minutes of vigorous cardio exercise still = 500 calories. Holy fat cow, no magic! You son of bitch Dale, you tricked me and told me I only needed to work out 25 minutes per day instead of 50 but you still want me to do it on 250 calories less per day. And 250 sounds like a lot of calories. Let's examine that theory for a minute. Two slices of bread on average is about 200 calories = Exercise for 30 minutes and eliminate two slices of bread per day = one pound of weight loss per week. One hamburger (no cheese) from McDonald's = 250 calories (cheeseburger = 300 calories). So 25 minutes of exercise and one less hamburger or cheeseburger per day = one pound of weight loss per week (actually if you eliminate the cheeseburger and reduce the exercise by five minutes). One glass of wine (8 oz) = 200 calories. Exercise for 30 minutes and eliminate one glass of wine (8 oz) = one pound of weight loss per week. This is getting easier by the second isn't it? I think you have the basics of my formula now and you can figure the rest out on your own and multiply it up. WARNING: You're obese – one pound per week isn't enough. Two pounds should be your minimum target per week. That's a 7,000 calorie per week deficit. Yes, that's going to be more work. It's going to be more exercise and more sacrifice. You will do it because you're worth it. Your skinny self wants out of this disgusting shell it's trapped inside of. Your skinny self is trapped in solitary confinement and can only see out through the eye holes of this massive cell you've encased them in. What did your skinny self do to deserve this imprisonment? Nothing! There may be a million physical, mental, psychological reasons you're imprisoning your skinny self, but this book is going to help that person escape the confines of your fat prison.

- One pound of fat = 3500 calories
- One minute of vigorous aerobic exercise = 10 calories (loss) per minute
    - **This level of fitness translates to one minute at 6.0 mph on a treadmill at a one percent incline**
    - If you are using a treadmill or elliptical or bike and not going this fast then you can adjust but the basic line above is where you need to be. I understand that as a fatty, 6.0 mph on a treadmill is a sprint. If you can only do 4.5 mph on the treadmill (3/4 of 6.0 mph) then you have to do 25 percent more than above ergo, 1:15 minutes to achieve that same 10 calories. Doesn't seem like much until you're an hour in and realize you have 15 minutes left. If you'd go faster it'd be over sooner. ☺
- One pound of weight loss per week = 500 calories per day deficit.
    - The best way to eliminate 500 calories per day is through a 50/50 combination of reducing the number of calories going in (reduce food intake) and increasing the number going out via exercise.

My other comment in the previous paragraph said 12 steps and Higher Power. I know that 10 - 20 percent of the people reading this book (possibly higher) have some type of addiction on the rainbow that I've previously mentioned throughout this book. Maybe it's alcohol, dysfunction, food, gambling, co-dependence, sex or love. If you are not already in a 12-step program you should seriously consider making that a part of your weight loss program. They are not quick fixes and they should not be taken or entered into lightly but they are probably a symptom of your obesity disease. You may not want to admit your addiction (we addicts call that the 1st of the 12 steps – that is, denial that is remedied by admitting that you are powerless over something that causes you harm in one way or another). Higher Power… Here's where I piss off some family and friends… Did I mention earlier in the book I was raised Catholic? Yes, good. I'm a devout agnostic so I embody the concept of a Higher Power. Some days my Higher Power is my running. Some days it's a man sitting on a cloud that looks like an old man with a long white beard. Some days it's a fat Asian man. Some days it's an elephant with eight arms. Some days it's little green men on a spaceship. Some days, it's me. Learn that you have a Higher Power and that they can help you achieve your goal.

Personal Trainer/Dietician – Again, if you're a fat beast these should not be negotiable things. You, most likely, may be incredibly motivated to which I give you a ton of credit, but take it from another fattie. You need help. You need professional help and are very unlikely to accomplish your goal without these two individuals in whatever form you can access them. I know I'm an extreme example. I know I had the means (money) to make this happen the right way. You may not have the means to make this happen, but there are alternative and creative ways to find help. You can look for programs from your town, city, or state. There are a ton of free programs everywhere to help you get started. I mentioned earlier that I don't endorse any particular plan like Weight Watchers or Jenny Craig or Curves but if it works for you, God's speed. Do it. These are great, often free programs. As for a personal trainer, go check your local YMCA and see if any of the personal trainers have any "friends" that train people as a side business. Check Craig's List – they're on there – just make sure they actually have certifications. Do not just start picking up weights and throwing them around. Do not just start a cardio program and think you're setting the world on fire and end up hurting yourself because you did too much too fast. Yes, you have to ramp up into any exercise program but done properly you can ramp up faster than you think, but you must ramp up and you must be consistent. **Consistency is key.** Having an appointment with a personal trainer or someone who's willing to help you is a strong driver to make sure you complete your assigned appointment.

Wow, it's wild to pull up some of my original spreadsheets to see where this journey started. As I told you above, I couldn't do it without a personal trainer. I tried. My original spreadsheet said I started this program with the intention of losing 50 pounds between September 18, 2010 and January 18, 2011. I had a plan. I wrote it down. It was a solid plan. I didn't do it until I got back from Key West in January 2011 lamenting over my "bitch tits." Damn it, I'm getting a personal trainer. Enter Chris G into my life. Here is the excerpt from my original spreadsheet log. I forget which beer I was drinking that was 136 calories each, but it was important enough for me to write down at the time. This was obviously before I went "on the wagon" for six months to reboot my system.

Goal = 50 lbs. loss between 9/18 and 1/18

Cardio - 3-4x per week (Treadmill, Elliptical, Cycle)
2 day - Cardio & AB
1 day - Cardio & AB & Weights (upper)
1 day - Cardio & AB & Weights (lower)

Legs - 2 sets 12 - 15 reps
Upper Body - 3 sets 12 - 15 reps

1 exercise for each body part

Need to eliminate 3,500 calories to = 1 lbs.
6 beers = 816 calories

When I first started working with my first trainer Chris G., he was strict, per my instructions, that our focus was losing weight; but he made sure that

I understood that while I'm losing all this weight we had to tighten/grow some muscle mass to fill out the skin/body that we'd be leaving behind. He helped sculpt me into what became the perfect vision of what I was asking for. I could not have asked for anything more than what Chris gave me. Our plan was a simple four to five days of cardio followed by a weight-training regimen that was primarily focused on "machines." I would always get to the gym an hour before our workouts so I could do 30 minutes of cardio which, as you can imagine, was BRUTAL in the beginning but got easier with experience and less weight. When people think of a gym or an exercise routine a cadre of different things come to their mind. Many people (I'd hazard to say most of you reading this) think of a Rocky-style gym with a boxing ring in the middle surrounded by "free weights" on racks, barbells, and benches where steroid-looking freaks are grunting and putting up more weight than your car could carry. Some people (I know some of you have actually been to a gym before) understand most gyms have this "free weight" component, but are mostly dominated by various types of "machines" whether they are circuit-based machines, resistance-based machines, or cardio-based machines. I think almost everyone has seen the classic treadmill, elliptical, bicycle-type machines.

Some think of it as merely a place to go do Yoga, Pilates, Zumba or other class based approaches to getting healthy. Maybe it's a P90X® or other modern version of group fitness where you jump up on boxes or join forces to flip tractor tires. The main point in this discussion is that the classic fattie is scared to walk into these places. I will help you overcome your fear. Everything in my approach included in this book has been a slow approach to getting you to accept the challenge that lies before you. You are chipping away at an iceberg with a tablespoon. It's slow, it's annoying in the beginning, but as you see the rapid progress you start to make at a certain point you get more and more invigorated to keep moving forward. You will develop (and this is my recommendation to you) tunnel vision when you go to the gym. Don't look at anyone or anything other than the Personal Trainer (PT) or Instructor. If you haven't sprung for a PT yet (what are you waiting for) you actually do want to look for a reasonably in-shape person who may be using a machine or lifting a particular weight as they are, hopefully, at least close to using the machine properly. Not always, which is why I still recommend you splurge in the beginning to get the PT, but if you just can't than make sure you don't hurt yourself doing any exercise as that will surely discourage you from continuing.

You MUST, SLOWLY, acclimate yourself to your new environment. This new "lifestyle" you are adopting WILL become the norm and a way of life. It must, you have no choice. I can officially say this as one of the people you know who goes to the gym and you hate me because I'm the "in shape" healthy guy. Guess what shit head? I was a slob just like you. You know what I think about your fatness now as I watch you walk into the gym and approach the treadmill like a cow walking the green mile towards the hamburger processing plant? I think, "You are a disgusting fat slob! BUT, at least you're here so you have my respect and I give you a ton (your weight) of credit for being here." Yes, that's what every in-shape, muscle-bound person at the gym thinks when you walk in. Sure you're disgusting. You know it. That's why you've made it this far in this book. But, damn it, you're going to change that. One day at a time, one week, one month, one quarter, one year at a time.

The new you will eventually see fat people walking into the gym and you will be the hated one who now thinks… "At least they're here." You'll offer them an encouraging smile and say "hi, glad you're here." As a runner I can tell you that EVERY runner I ever pass on A1A in Florida or when I was trail running in New Jersey ALWAYS said, "Good morning," "Hi," "Hello," "What a great day to be outside," "Nice day for a run," or at a minimum (if they were heavy into the miles or their music) they'd ALWAYS give at least a head nod or wave of the hand to indicate; "You're doing it. You're out here, being healthy, welcome to the club. It's an awesome club to be a member of." It takes six weeks to develop a habit (scientific fact). Start working out, going to the gym AT LEAST three days per week for six weeks. After six weeks, if you miss a day you will feel guilty and want to make up for it by going a fourth day. You'll feel so good after doing it for four days that particular week you may start going four days per week on a regular basis. Then, you caught it;

you caught the "healthy living fever". It's a good fever to catch. You will catch it. You must, you have no choice.

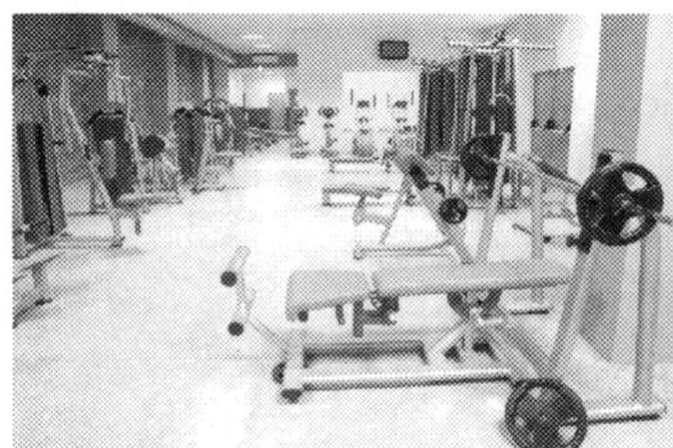
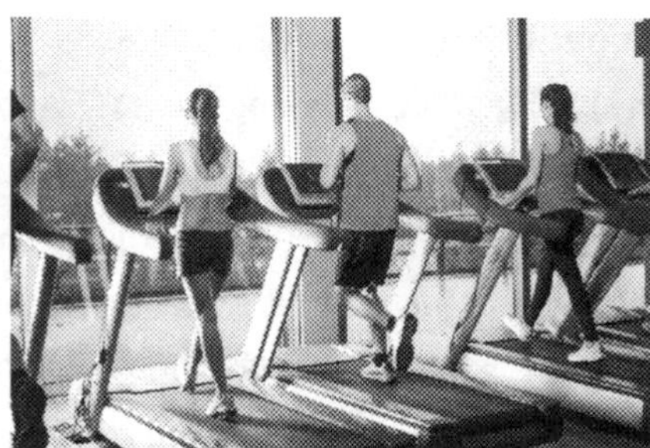

You know another area I feared when I first started getting healthy and going to a gym? Sweating! I hated to sweat. My girlfriend at the time and I used to have a running joke because she was very into healthy living (not sure why she was with a fat slob like me) that every time she came home from the gym I would insist that she "dispatch with the stink cells forthwithly." As she was in the shower I would ask, "Are you using a lot of soap." She'd always answer in that kid-type whining tone, "Yeeeeesssss." "Well use more," I'd shout! I would even occasionally sneak into the bathroom while she was showering and squirt some liquid soap over the shower curtain to make sure she was using enough. Again, I have practical good advice here that many of you haters/doubters will resist at first. Trust a fellow fattie. I KNOW WHAT I'M TALKING ABOUT BROTHER/SISTER! While I wouldn't say that I've learned to love sweating, I've learned that every drop of sweat that comes out of me represents my flowing journey on this healthy path. So I'm acclimating to sweat. My analogy MAY be lost on people who's ideal vacation is skiing in the Rockies or the Alps or traveling in the Arctic circles, but stick with me for a minute and you'll be able to relate my approach for desensitization to your world in one way or another.

For me to get used to sweating I had to place myself in the mental state that I was on vacation on a Caribbean island or a beach in Florida where it was in the 90s with a relatively high humidity. To replicate this in the gym I would do my cardio (that would get that first layer of sweat going). Then I would do my weight or other circuit training (that wouldn't produce as much sweat as the cardio) but it wouldn't stop it, either. Finally, when I was ready to stretch it out or "cool down" I would do my stretching or "cool down" in the gym's sauna/spa/steam room (whichever was available to me based on where I was). When I was looking for a gym to join this was an important factor for me. Your gym doesn't have one? Find a "hot yoga" class to take once a week. Turn up the heat excessively high in your home before you leave for the gym so by the time you get home you can stretch on your floor in your own "hot house." It's all doable and practical. When you put yourself in the mindset of sweating on a beach somewhere you will also begin to associate the workout with a pleasurable experience. Again, it's going to take time. Create your own scenario where you project mental imagery of a calm, relaxed, warm/ hot environment where you can associate the workout you just did (and the associated sweating) with a tranquil, peaceful, relaxed environment.

A friend asked me one of the ways I stay motivated. The following is an excerpt of an email I sent to her. I have found the best way for me is twofold and I know it will work for most people. Thirty pounds on a woman can be gone in three - six months without being too radical. The twofold approach to staying motivated is Goal Timing and Publicity. The two ways to really lose the weight and keep it off are: 1) Use my Goal method below and 2) Determine your demon and detox from it. What's your demon? Mine was alcohol. I had to give it up "cold turkey" for six months to "reboot" my body. It's goal motivation. Set a goal! Do it today. Here's a hint... Go to www.active.com. Find a 5K run that's three months away. PLENTY of time! Pay $20 (or whatever it costs), and sign up for this 5K. It doesn't matter if you run, run/walk, walk it, or crawl. IT DOESN'T MATTER! JUST SIGN UP FOR THE GODDAMNED RACE, TRAIN FOR IT, SHOW UP, AND DO IT! After you sign up I want you to tell EVERYONE (did you hear me – I said - **EVERYONE**) you know that you're doing it. Tell your friends, family, co-workers, spouse, your social groups (church, etc...). Put it on LinkedIn, Facebook, Twitter, etc...Be public about you doing a 5K and be proud of it. Damn it – you're a healthy person you should be proud of it and you're supporting a good cause (whatever the 5K is sponsoring). Finishing is winning. Screw time if it's your first one. You did 3.1 miles. That's more than that fat slobbo of a friend of yours can do. What'll be even more empowering is that it's even more than that skinny, blond bitch at work can do. She's never done a 5K before (it'd be tough in six-inch stilettos anyway).

Once you finish this 5K (no matter how you cross the line) you will want to do it again and you will do it again and you'll be public about it (again) and you will get faster (doesn't matter if it's walking faster - you'll get faster). Soon, you'll entertain the thought of a 10K and then maybe even a half marathon and then someday (it took me three years) before I finally said, OK, I've got this 5K, 10K, 15K, and half marathon thing down. I've run 18 miles (again – took me over two years to get to that point) I think I have 26.2 miles in me. I followed the same advice I mentioned above. To quote the Godfather movie… "I want it public and I want it messy." Smear yourself and your race goal. Don't back off, do it right, train appropriately and accomplish your goal. If you choose to do a bike race, a rowing race, a swim event, a biathlon, or a triathlon, all of the same rules apply. Commit, advertise, train, accomplish, promote, pat yourself on the back for being awesome, and do it again.

The following exercises where written down and dictated to me by my two PTs (both Chris G and Kevin K). In the beginning Chris G's approach was to help me lose weight and add some muscle to compensate and supplement to newer healthier Dale. Once Kevin got a hold of the healthier, fitter, skinnier Dale, he wanted to mold an image of himself. This skinny Dale could be as much of an athlete as Kevin and Dale doesn't even know it. Kevin replaced many, but not all, of the weight- lifting exercises I was doing with more functional-type exercises. That is, fewer machines and more body weight and natural movement exercises. It wasn't better than what Chris G had done for me, it was just different and more appropriate for the healthy, fit, athlete I was becoming. Both were necessary steps in my personal development.

The first set of exercises was primarily what Chris G had me focus on for the first year. The second set is what I switched to once Kevin K entered the picture. The first set of exercises is broken down into the following categories: Back, Biceps, Chest, Core, Legs, Shoulders, and Triceps. The second sets of exercises (Kevin's more functional type exercises) are broken into: Lower, Upper, Core, Triceps, Biceps, and Core. Yes, I said "core" three times. Probably still isn't enough but both PTs were supporting my newfound love of running. Whatever form of cardio you have or will adopt as a result of this book will be developed and enhanced by the building of your core.

What you should take away from this list is NOT a recipe but suggested ingredients in your weight-loss formula. No one exercise or even set of exercises will lead to you dropping the pounds within the overall commitment to healthy living including your cardio, cardio, cardio that will continue in conjunction with the exercises below.

Remember, I was doing an average of four days per week of intense cardio and then two days of weight training. If I could fit in a fifth day or cardio, I would reserve the exercises for that day to be strictly core and abdominal work because those exercises are quicker in the grand scheme than upper or lower type exercises (be they functional or weight specific). I know you have many questions. I would, too, if I was as fat as you and was reading this like it was Greek. Oh that's right! I was as fat as you or fatter. AND, I did it, I learned, I improved, SLOWLY, but I improved. It was hard, it was long, and it was a commitment. There is no better commitment you can make to yourself in your entire life than to get and remain healthy. It doesn't matter what other issues or problems you have. They are all easier to tackle, cope with, and conquer if you are physically and psychologically stronger. I can and will help you with the physical part. The psychological part – I'll try but that's not my goal here.

So, you have myriad of questions… When do I do cardio? When do I do the weight training? How much weight should I be using so as not to hurt myself but have the most impact? Should I do them on the same day? Which should I do first? Holy shit, how long were you at the gym? Were you really there five – six days per week? How many hours a week did you spend doing this? You told me in the beginning of this book I only needed to give you 24 minutes a day. WTF? Did you lie to me?

Personal Trainer

I will sum up the answer to all these questions in two words, but I will then explain it in-depth in simple terms that even a butterball like you will understand. I know you're going to throw another fit when I give you the two words, but please just keep reading. If you have to throw something, curse me out, hit your spouse (kidding – don't do that), kick the dog (I'd rather you hit your spouse then kick the dog), spank your children (better than the spouse or the dog because they probably did something to deserve it – you just don't know it yet) then you should do that and get it out of your system; and then come back and keep reading what's AFTER those two words. Here are your two words… In the context of a book I'm going to whisper them, and then I'll repeat them a little louder, and then if you're hard of hearing, I will yell them to you… The two-word answer to all your questions above (and the ones I forgot to list) is: Personal Trainer, let me say it a little louder; Personal Trainer, did you hear it that time? No, OK, one more time. **PERSONAL TRAINER!** I saw it. I saw the vein in your head or neck pop out. Here are four simple facts: If I want to know if this lump in my scrotum is cancer I can ask my co-worker or I can go see a doctor. If I need to change the transmission in my car I can call my drunken cousin Skeeter (I apologize if you really have a cousin named Skeeter) or I can take it to a reputable mechanic. If I am anorexic and I want to gain weight (and a lot of it and quickly) I would ask, well, I'd ask you. If I want to do exercises, properly, not hurt myself, and achieve the most benefit in the shortest amount of time I would ask a Personal Trainer… Here's the ton of disclaimers. I do not have a personal training certificate (yet). I am not endorsed nor will I probably ever be by any of the personal trainer certifying bodies (not that I don't want to be in case they read this and want to make me a paid spokesperson). I just fundamentally believe that if you could do this yourself you would have done it by now, but you're still fat so you haven't and you can't do it by yourself. Admitting that you are powerless over your fat addiction is a noble first step. Asking for help from your Higher Power or a certified Personal Trainer is a great second step. I'm not purposely putting you down but you're stupid, you got fat, it happens, we're Americans or living in America. It's one of the many reasons the rest of the world hates us so much. We are an obese society. It's in our culture. We believe we've earned it. Well, my friend, the time has come to pay the piper or soon you'll be paying the ferryman to take you across the river.

The exercises below may or may not have comments next to them, but I will attempt to say something about each one. If it's blank, it's because the exercise is probably self-evident; and while it was part of my routine, it didn't really leave a lasting impact on my memory … at least not enough for me to comment on.

You're going to ask me what the different muscles are: See the pictures below if you have questions. If a particular muscle is not on here than Google's not too far away.

Muscle Groups

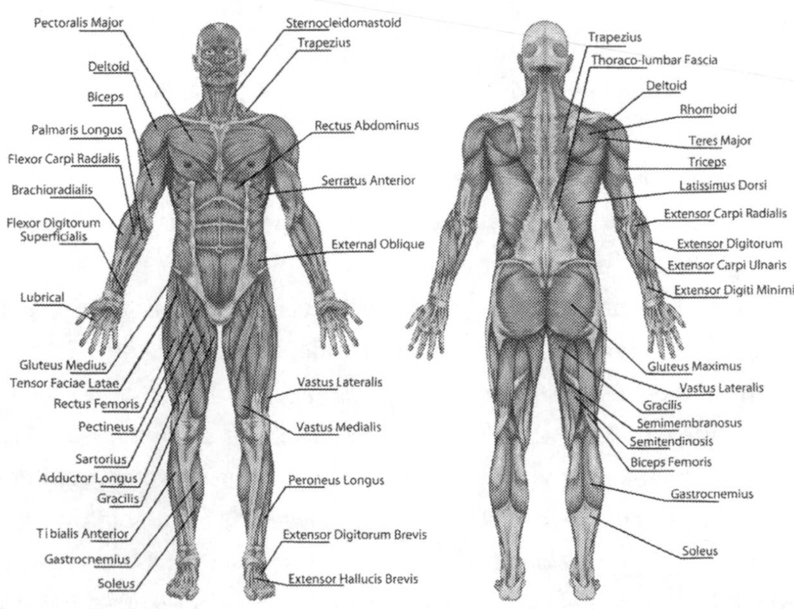

If there are any particulars that I need to point out I will include them in this paragraph. Throughout some of the exercises you may see S-____, C-____. These referred to seat or chest placements. Every resistance or weight machine (besides free weights) probably has some type of adjustment that you can set so you are doing the exercise properly (you won't know unless you have a PT). Each exercise obviously has a focus area. On one day (of my two weight-training days) I would work out either upper or lower and back or core. That's possible combinations or upper/back, upper/core, lower/back, lower/core. Triceps, Biceps, and Shoulders are obviously upper. Back, Core, and Chest are core. Some would consider chest to be "upper" but it doesn't really matter where you slot it as long as you incorporate it into your routine. DB stands for dumb bell. No, that's not me being a smart ass referring to your partner or spouse. DBs are the "small" free weights usually made of steel, lead, or plastic with something inside like concrete or other material.

They vary in weight from one pound up to 60+. All resistance/weight exercises should be done a certain number of times (this is called repetitions or reps). Typical reps vary from 8 – 15 but usually fall somewhere in the middle, that is, 10 – 12. Typically, the lighter the weight you are using the higher your reps should be for the individual exercise. A set of 12 reps should typically be done three times or three sets of reps. Typically, between each set is a recovery period of 30 – 90 seconds where you're giving your muscles enough time to stop pulsating, but only enough to allow you to do the next set with the same efficiency as the previous set. Of course, there are a ton of different types of rep / set combinations including those without recovery time, those with significantly more reps, those with one or two reps that have a significantly higher weight associated with the exercise. No two programs are alike, nor should they be. Your PT should customize your workout to your goals and to your body and or issues. Anything less is doing you a disservice and may even risk injury. You need to know your limits but at the same time you need to push yourself. You're going to continue the excuses. That's what fatties like you do. Shut the hell up and deal with the little pain. Pain is weakness leaving the body. No pain, no gain. Part of training is injury. While technically, these are euphemistic statements they are true to some extent.

Every time you doing something like strength training or cardio like running you are tearing the muscles apart to allow them to rebuild themselves and make themselves stronger. So, with this, I present the initial set of exercises in no particular order that I utilized with my PT to help get rid of my initial weight (approximately 70 pounds). Not all gyms will have all this equipment but a good PT will be able to use the machines that they have to perform the exercises below so bring the book, show them the picture and have fun working out. You are going to feel so good (after the 3rd day) ☺.

Exercise Reference Chart

Exercise	Focus Area	Comment
Biangular Lat Row Also called "Low Row" S-____, C-____	Back	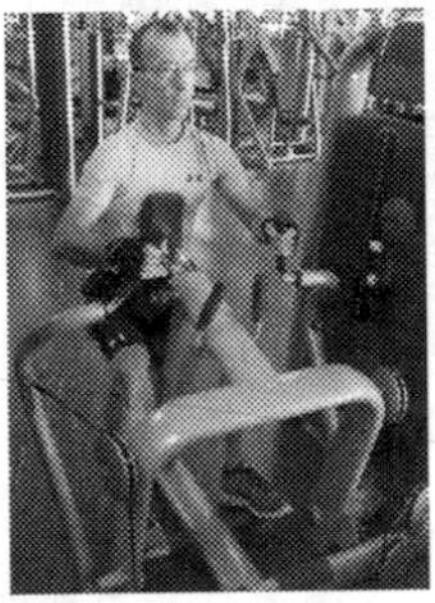 Need to set the seat and chest to make sure your arms are extended with just a slight bend in the elbows. Pulling back keeping the elbows close to the chest. Squeeze those lat muscles
DB bent rows	Back	Good exercise that can be done anywhere with any weight. Can be done with a resistance band. I found, when I was traveling for work these were the types of exercises that came in handy because many hotel gyms are so crappy you need easy things you can do while you're away from your home gym.

Gravitron Pull-Ups Wide	Back	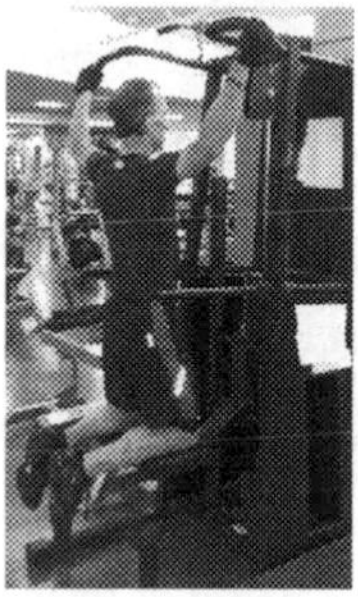 Hard to describe the machine without showing it but once you see it you know what it is. Great machine for switching between assisted pull ups and tricep dips. If you can't do a pull up to save your life (like me – even now that I'm healthy) these "assisted" pull ups give you strength and self-confidence. The picture shows someone doing pull ups but this machine can also do tricep dips if you grab the lower handles in the same manner and push up.
Hyperextensions	Back	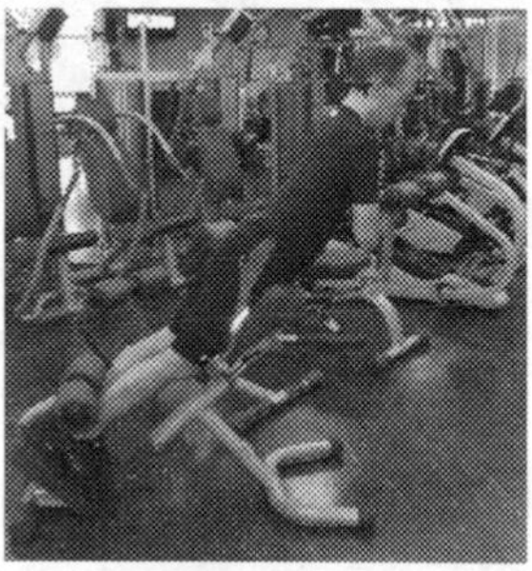 One of the most basic things you see at the gym and you probably never knew what it was. I certainly didn't. When I was fat I was always worried I was going to tip it over so I had Chris or Kevin keep a foot on the back or tossed a 40 pound steel plate on the back legs. It was because my gut was so big it weighted the machine forward. Eventually, I found I could hold a weight to my chest to make this more challenging. GREAT to stretch and strength your lower back (lumbar) muscles.

Inverted rows	Back	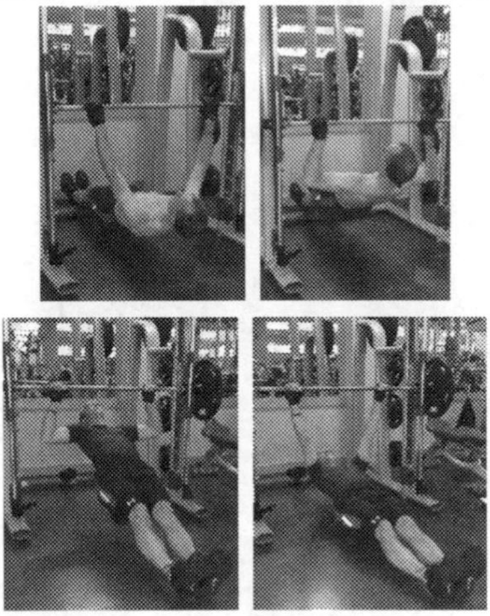 I had to show both the front and back view of this simple exercise. Simple. Yeah, you can ask Chris G. This exercise was the anti-Christ of my journey to strength training. I absolutely HATED these. I said earlier I can't do a pull up/ chin up. What would make you think I could do them from a lying position any easier? Truth be told, my back, lats, and chest are partially what they are today thanks to these. Whenever I'm in a mood to torture myself I still do these. Great with the TRX bands as well.
Lat Pull Down	Back	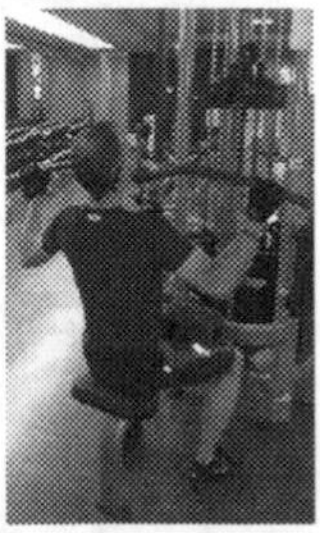 Pretty simple exercise. I learned the hard way however that if the weight stack is on the side (the picture here shows the weight in the center) do not lean over to change the weight to something higher unless the machine is bolted to the floor. You'd be surprised how easy it is for a fat bastard like you (or me) to tip one of these things over and look like an ass when you have to help the trainer pick up about 1,000 pounds of machine off of your own hand. I have that scar/battle wound to this day.

Nautilus Lower Back	Back	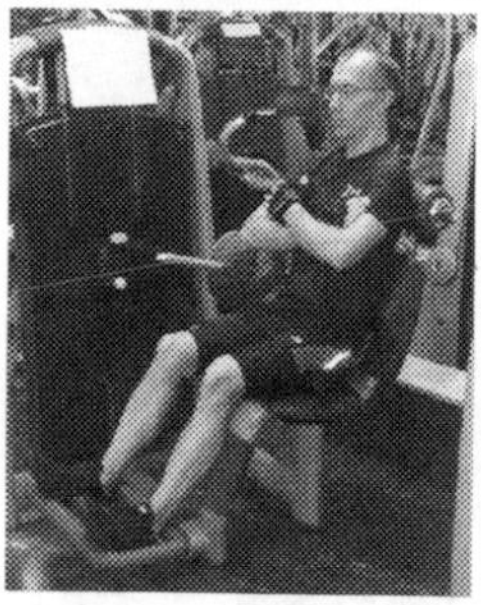 Old standby. I did this exercise almost every workout. Fantastic for lumbar. Why do I do so many lumbar exercises…? This may be more important for the men than the women but when you have a beer gut like I had and all the strain of that belly is transferred to your back, it's very easy to hurt your back while you're jogging/running and losing all that weight. It's a good idea to keep that back nice and strong, which is only going to prevent other running injuries as well.
Bicep Zottman	Biceps	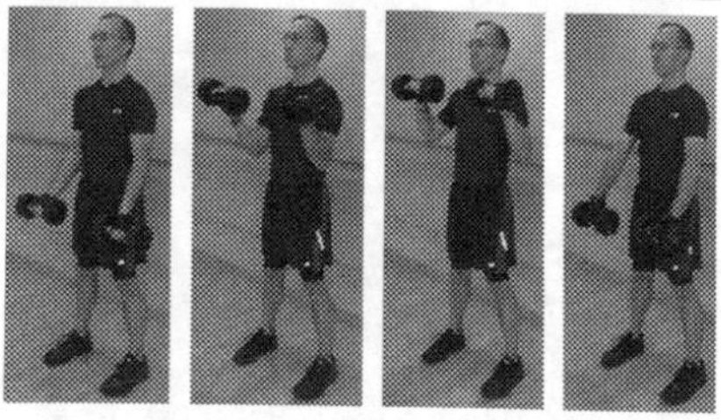 Another great exercise if you're on the road and can only grab a pair of dumb bells. 4 motions, standard bicep curl, turn wrists away and lower back down slowly. Use enough weight to make it difficult.
Biceps Cable Curls	Biceps	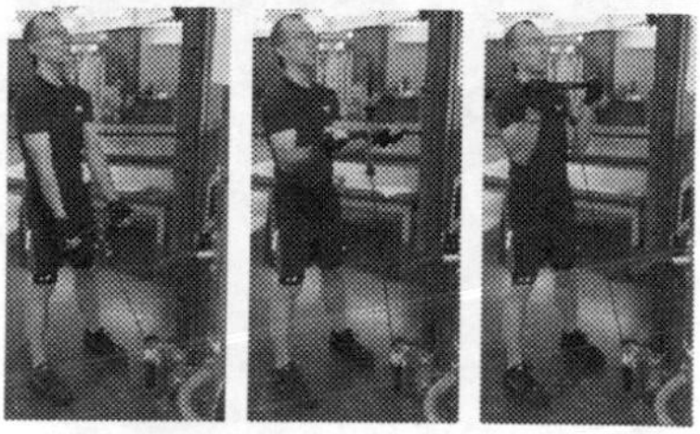 Pretty basic. Not much to say here. They're good, do them.

Preacher DB	Biceps	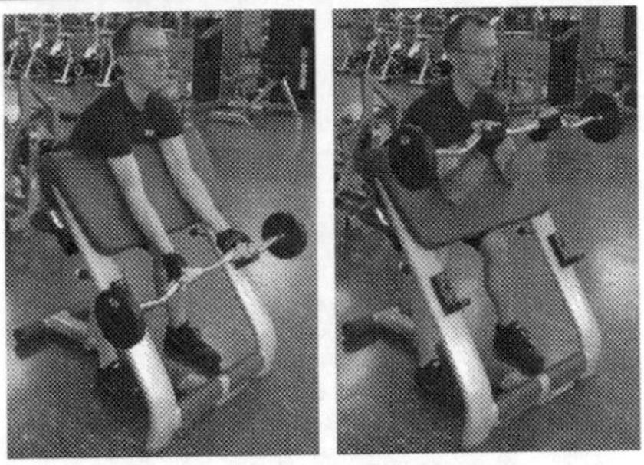 Again, pretty basic but another bench you may have seen at the gym and never really knew what it was used for. A worthy exercise but good to have a spotter/PT make sure you're pulling it correctly.
Rope curls	Biceps	Almost exactly the same as the Cable Curls listed above except instead of using the bar in the picture above you use the large rope. If you've seen the rope next to the machine you know what I'm talking about. If you're not sure just do the one above. This is a slight variation to keep it interesting.
Chest Press	Chest	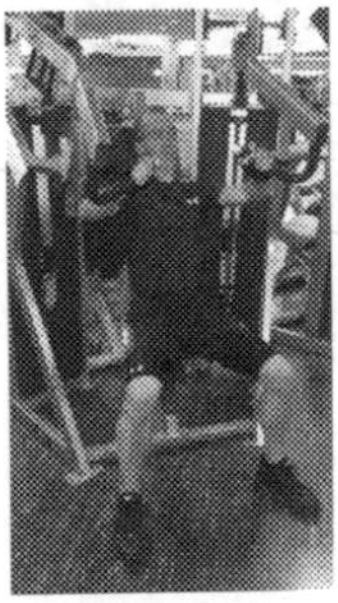 Very basic machine – couldn't be more important for ridding yourself of those bitch tits guys. Ladies – you want the girls to be a little firmer (yeah, do these).

Flat bench	Chest	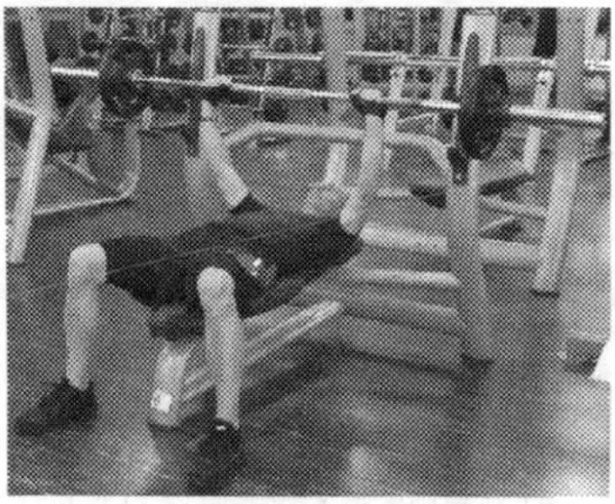 The classic image of the free weight guy in the gym. Possibly visions of Rocky come to mind. **Important:** do not attempt this exercise without a spotter or PT. If you have never used free weights before you must get instruction from someone who knows what they're talking about before attempting these. I will refer below to how you can do this similar exercise with dumb bells. Using DB is not a bad way to ease into this critical chest exercise.
Gravitron Dips	Chest	See the Gravitron pull-ups listed above. These are the opposite. Instead of hanging on the top bar and pulling yourself up. You are grabbing the lower bars and lowering yourself down until your forearms are at a 90 degree angle and then back up. You should be able to use the same "assist" weight (or close to it) as the pull ups.
Incline DB press	Chest	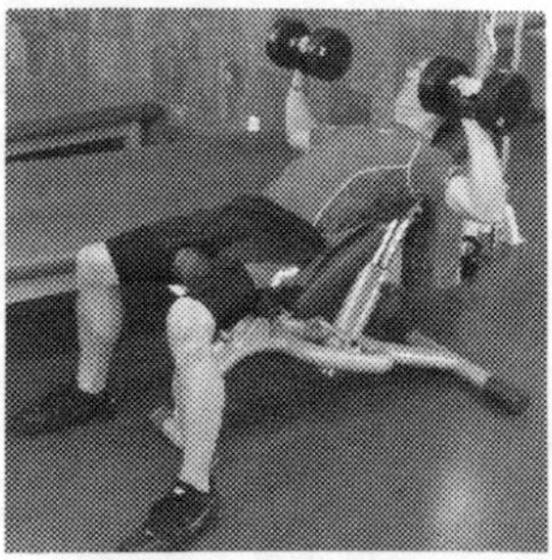 This is a good way to slowly introduce yourself to the flat chest bench press. The only thing to be careful with here is when you are complete you should rock forward to place the DB in front of you as opposed to letting your arms unnaturally fall to the sides and potentially hurt or pull something.

Pectoral Fly S-____, P-____	Chest	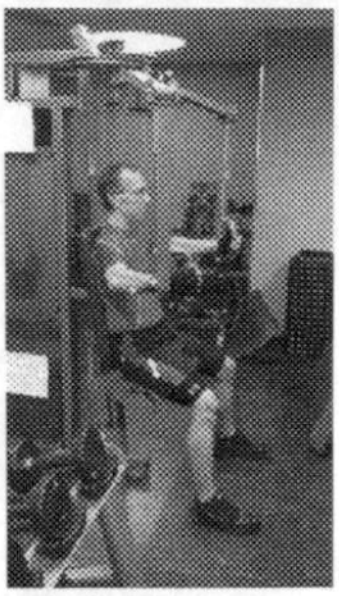 Another oldie but a goodie. These are also so important for both guys and women. Visualize your chest muscles bringing the arms of the machine together. Don't forget to set the seat to the proper height. Align your hands (with a slight bend in the elbow) at about the same level as your nipples. The P is the Pin setting (if there is one) on where the handles start. Start perfectly with your arms at 180 degrees. You only have to go back about 160 degrees on recoil but tell a PT to correct your form.
Push-ups	Chest	The classic favorite (NOT). For ladies you can keep your knees on the ground with feet crossed to make this a little easier.
Crunches w/ med ball	Core	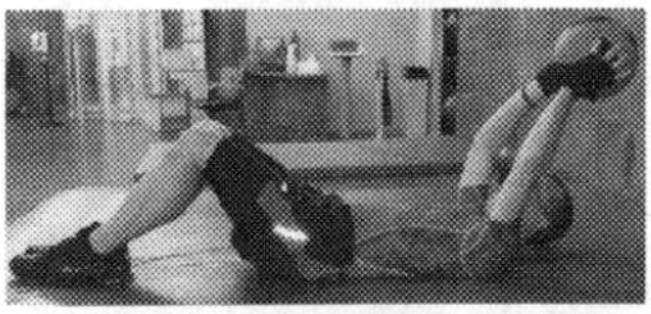 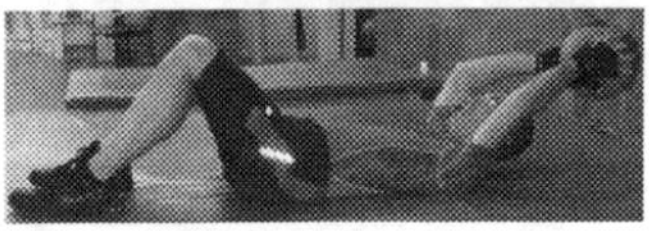 Notice that the movement is not that big, so don't be afraid to use a heavier medicine ball than you think. At least 12 lbs. for men and 8 lbs. for women

Leg Lifts / Planks	Core	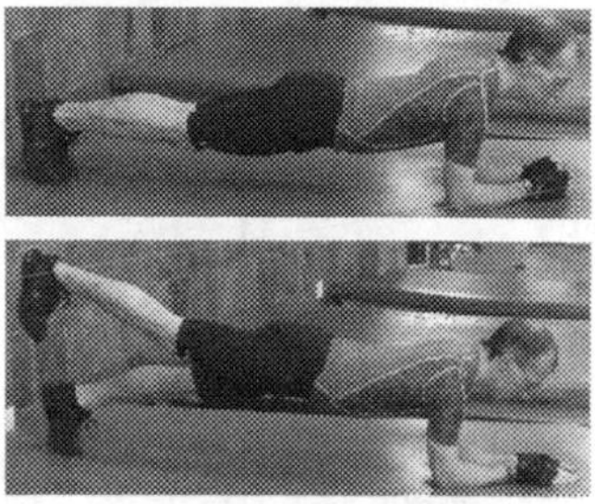 Regular plank on the left and a plan with a raised leg on the right. Either should be held and or repeated. Start with holding it for 3 x 30 seconds and work up to 3 x 60 seconds with 50 percent of that time as a rest. Of course, if you're adding leg lifts make sure you do both sides.
Oblique ball toss	Core	This one is tough to do if your gym doesn't have a racquetball court or isn't fond of you scaring the hell out of the people playing racquetball on the next court. The object is to throw the medicine ball using your side oblique's to propel the ball high enough to be able to catch it as it bounces off the wall. This can work with a partner but you will be limited by the person's ability to catch and re-throw the ball to you in a timely fashion. And, when it's a wall instead of another person it allows you to take out more frustrations.
Torso Rotations	Core	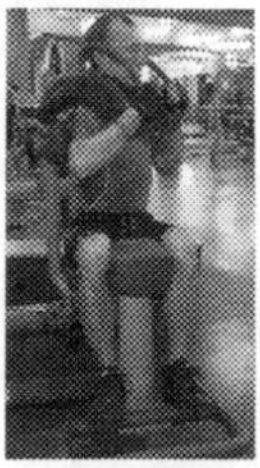 Most people probably aren't sure what that funny looking machine does that people sit on and twist from side to side. AND, for that reason I will not even begin to describe in this book how to use it. Ask. It's a great machine when used properly with the proper amount of weight and movement. You should include it as it's AWESOME for the love handles but you need to do it right so you don't tweak your back. Ask, don't be afraid to ask the local PT for the proper form while using this machine.

Abductor (Outer)	Legs	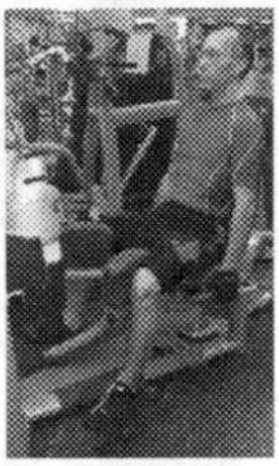 Sorry ladies, while men typically refer to these exercises as feminine or by other rude names like vagina exercises they are far from and they are critical exercises for both men and women because this is one of the muscles we don't often work unless we're ballerina's or runners. As a runner it is critical to work these muscles because they will help your stride. Notice the difference as they both, sometimes, use the same machine. In one case the pads are outside the knees and you are pushing against them and in the other case the pads are inside the knees and you are squeezing them. Again, both critical and they should be done together in sets since you're using the machine anyway.
Adductor (Inner)	Legs	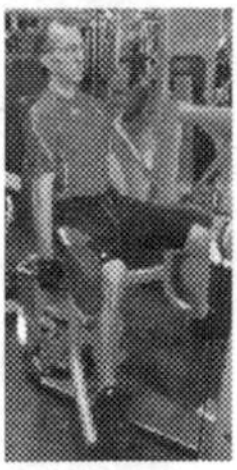 See above – same applies. In this case I am demonstrating using two different machines, sometimes it's the same machine.
BWS	Legs	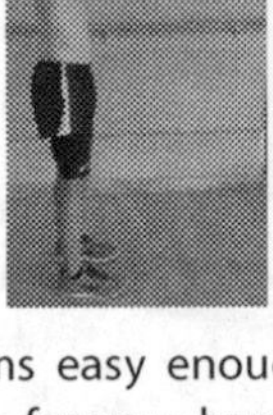 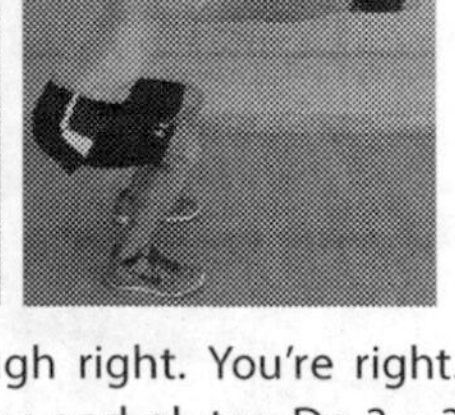 Seems easy enough right. You're right. Do them for your hams and glutes. Do 3 x 30 at a shot.

Front squats	Legs	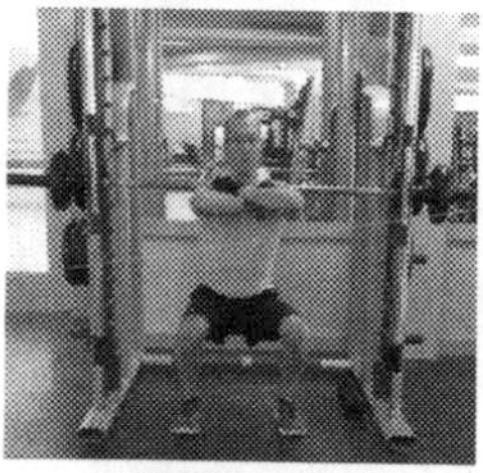 Yes, that is what it looks like. A barbell balancing on your biceps and shoulders while you loosely grab onto it and do a squat (similar to above) without putting your hands out (that is, don't let go of the bar. Weight can be just the bar itself or you can start with only 2.5 lbs on each side. Either way, this is another exercise to be careful with and make sure you have a spotter (that is a PT) to make sure your form is correct. You can also use the Smith machine as shown.
Glute/Ham	Legs	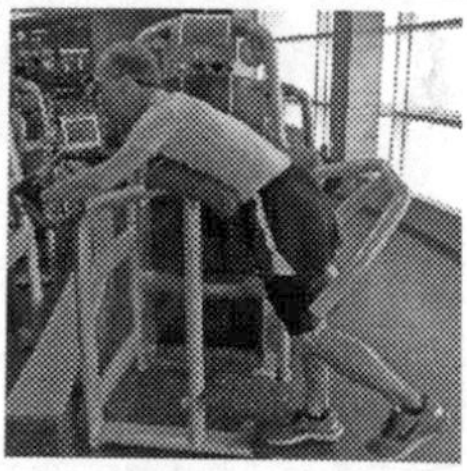 These are also called kickbacks because that's exactly what you are doing as you are leaning forward on the machine. You are kicking back with one leg while the other knee rests on the pad. They look deceptively easy but you quickly realize that you don't need much weight to make these exercises difficult. 10 – 20 pounds is probably enough to make you realize that you've never really worked out your glutes.

Leg Extension (Quad)	Legs	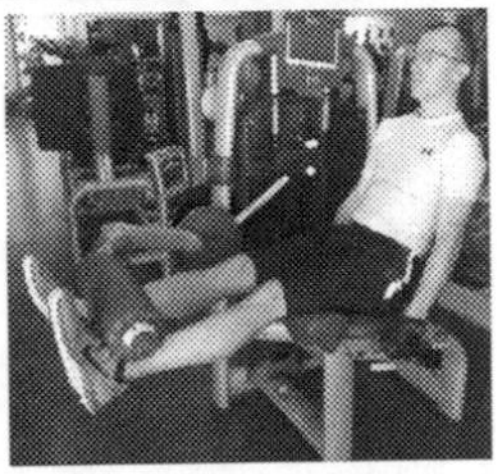 One of the more basic machines at the gym but definitely one you should be using. Moderate weight can be applied and yes, even if you're a runner you can incorporate these into your routine, especially if you're trying to lose weight at the same time.
Leg/Toe Press	Legs	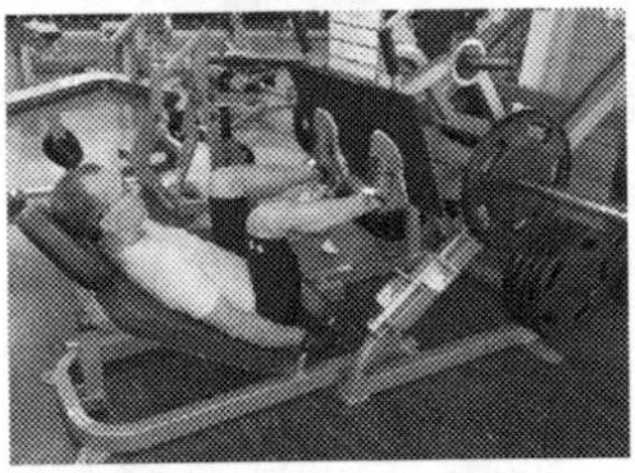 This machine is obviously used for both leg pressing as well as toe presses. It's shown again below.
Lying Leg Curl (Ham) 2 holes out	Legs	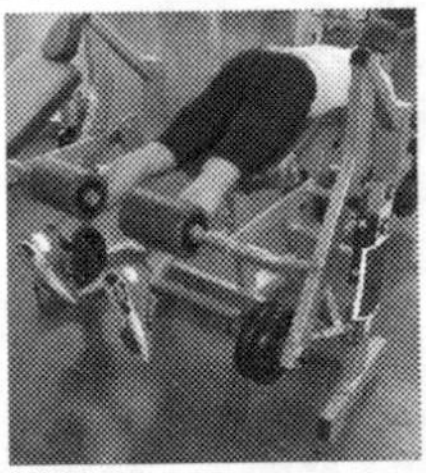 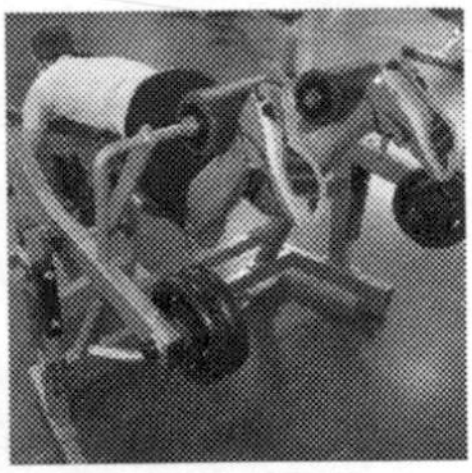 This one looks uncomfortable and the first few times you will probably feel that way. Once you've burned your hams into submission they will thank you. This reminds me, I need to do more of these. As a runner we often neglect working our hams.
PL leg press	Legs	PL stands for Plate Loaded. Whenever you see those letters in these exercises it's referring to that type of machine where you actually have to lift plates onto the machine instead of just moving a pin from one hole to another. Shown above as well but for working quads and hams, there is no better machine to build some muscle while burning some fat simultaneously.

Seated Calf Raise	Legs	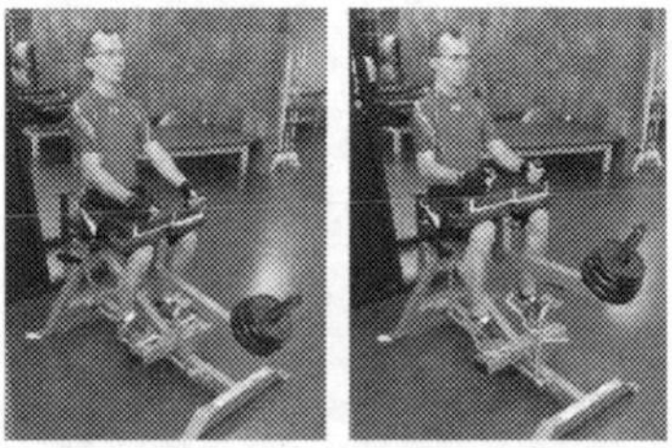 Wow, now that I'm running longer distances I REALLY need to do more of these. We need to keep that Achilles muscle stretched. So easy to injure and get stiff. When you get out of bed in the morning and you feel like your ankles are a hinge joint that need oil to unlock them this means you're not doing enough calf/toe raises.
Seated Leg Curl (Ham) S-2, A-2, 2 showing	Legs	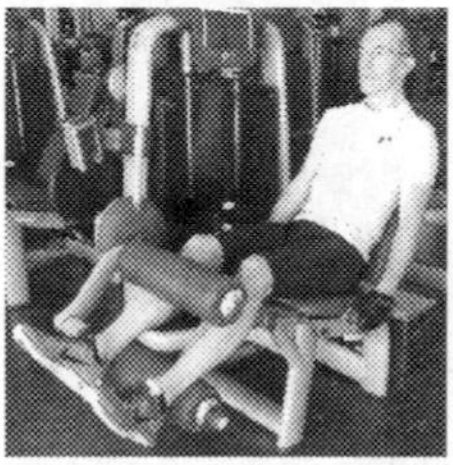 As shown. Pretty basic. Moderate weight. Another good ham exercise. Trying to show different variations of exercises so you don't get bored.
Walking lunges	Legs	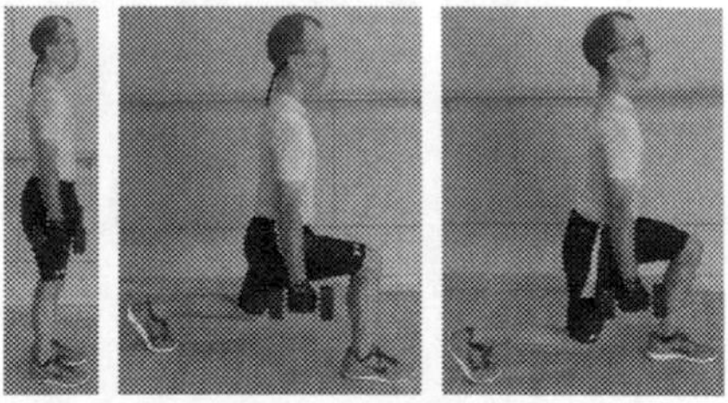 Sorry, I know they suck. I know they look easy. You can do them standing in place or walk a straight line but make sure you have a dumbbell in each hand. Doesn't need to be much 5 – 10 for women and 10 – 25 for men. Should be about twice the weight of the suitcase or briefcase or other tool you may carry for a living.

DB side laterals	Should	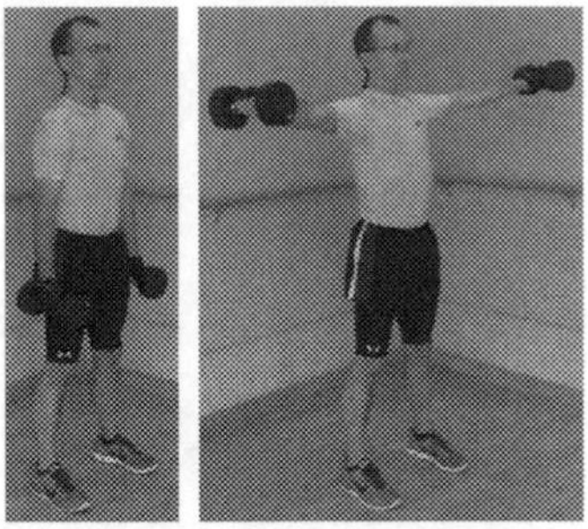 Since my MBA was done at St. Joseph's University in Philadelphia I often refer to these exercises as the ones our school mascot must be able to do a million. Light to moderate weight and flap those arms like a bird with a slight bend in the elbow.
One arm DB press	Should	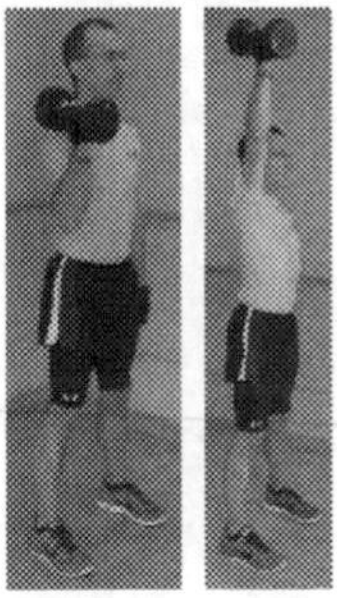 Pretty basic. Low to moderate weight. Basic shoulder exercise but worth incorporating into your regular workout.
Shoulder Press	Should	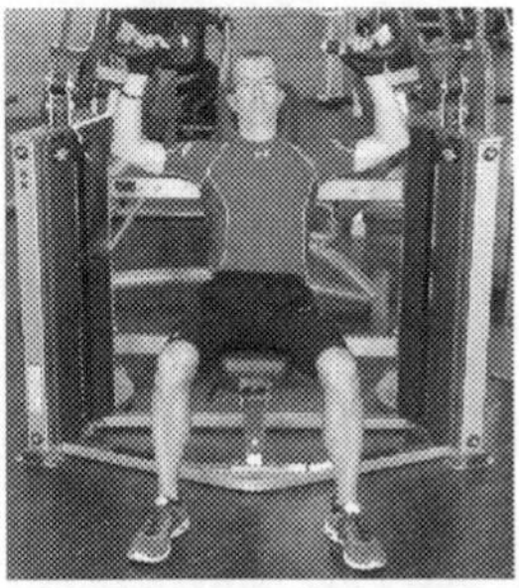 Another one of the basic machines in the gym that must be used as a regular part of your shoulder routine.

Shrugs (Traps)	Should	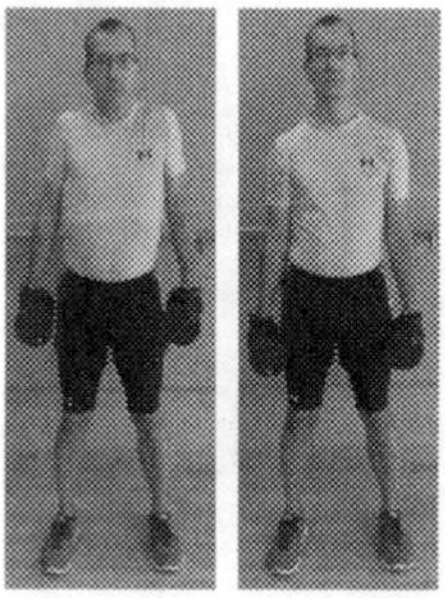 Not sure if the picture does this justice but it's a very easy exercise. Dumbbell in each hand. Lift your shoulders straight up. I used to laugh when I was doing these because my PT taught me to do them like I was talking to my girlfriend at the time. "So what do you want to do this weekend?" I would do the shrug and say to myself, "I dunno," "I dunno," "I dunno," "I dunno," "I dunno," 15 times. It was silly but it made me laugh and if that's what gets you through the exercise then so be it.
One arm DB ext _Tricep	Tricep	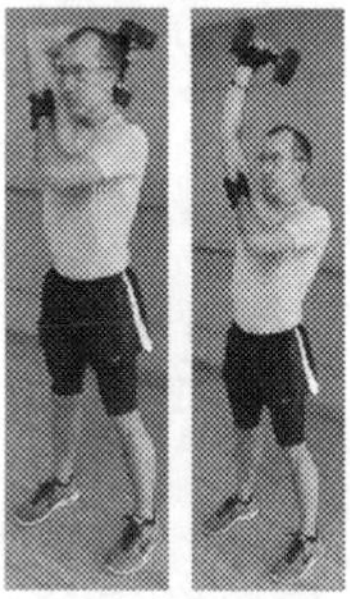 The "first" time I saw these I thought they "looked" easy. Holy shit was my tricep hurting for the week afterwards. What's most surprising to me is that you're supposed to use a moderate amount of weight here. At least 10 – 12 for women and 15 – 25 for men or more. You should hold the arm raising the weight with the other hand as shown to make sure your form is correct and that you're raising the dumbbell directly overhead and bending the elbow to a 90 degree angle back down so the weight is completely behind your head.

One arm reverse pushdown	Tricep	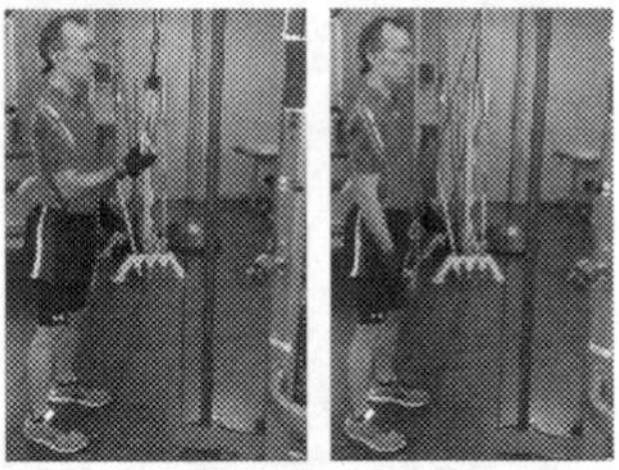 Never knew of a reason to use the machine or the big thing standing there with the cables on it? Well, you do now. For this and the next exercise. For this one, you can use one hand and pull the cable and weight down.
Tri PushDown Vbar	Tricep	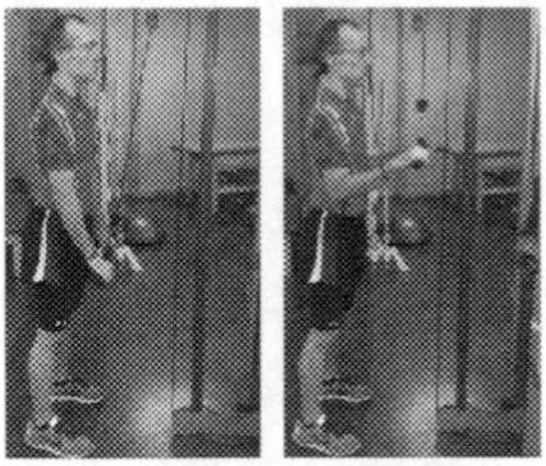 This motion is similar to the one above except that you are using the bar (the one with the V's in it) and gripping it with both hands and pulling it down.
Triceps (Skullcrusher)	Tricep	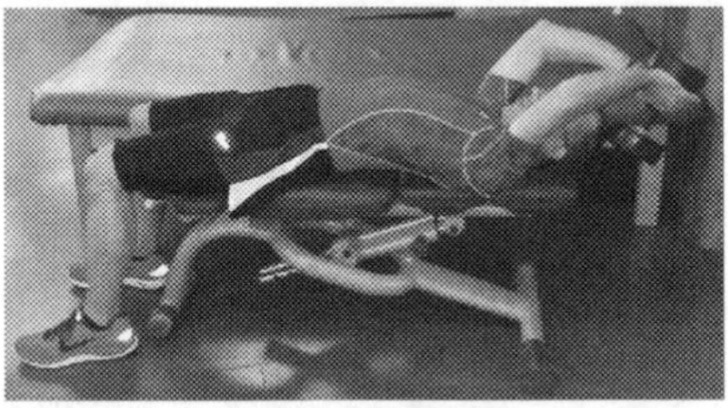 Just what they sound like. Don't drop the dumbbell. It hurts. I can testify that it will leave a bump, make you see stars, and make you think your ex is the most beautiful person on earth. OK, maybe not the last one but don't drop it. Use two hands and lower the dumbbell behind your head. It may or may not be obvious but you should be using a decent-size dumbbell for this exercise. More incentive not to drop it.

The next sets of exercises are the functional exercises, primarily used by my second PT, Kevin. Many of the exercises below were also listed above and if that's the case then I will simply refer back to the previous section. My point of listing them twice is to show my beginning stages of "getting healthy" with my first PT, Chris, and then my continued training with the person who served as my volunteer running coach and then became my official PT once Chris moved to South Florida. Once I saw how much overlap there was between the two sections I seriously thought about deleting the duplicate rows but I decided to include them to show the overlap and why some of these exercises were judged by my running coach to be just as important as some of the previous areas focused on by my previous PT. It also reflects my overall increased level of fitness and ability to handle "bigger boys" exercises.

Exercise	Focus Area	Comment
Front Squats	Lower	Described on previous pages.
PL Leg Press	Lower	Described on previous pages.
Glute/Ham	Lower	Described on previous pages.
Lying Leg Curl (Ham)	Lower	Described on previous pages.
Abductor (Outer)	Lower	Described on previous pages.
Adductor (Inner)	Lower	Described on previous pages.
Seated Calf Raise	Lower	Described on previous pages.
Toe Press / Leg Press	Lower	Described on previous pages.

Flat bench	Upper	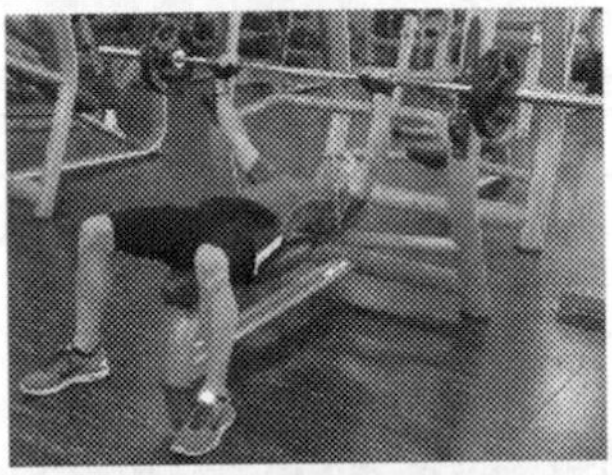 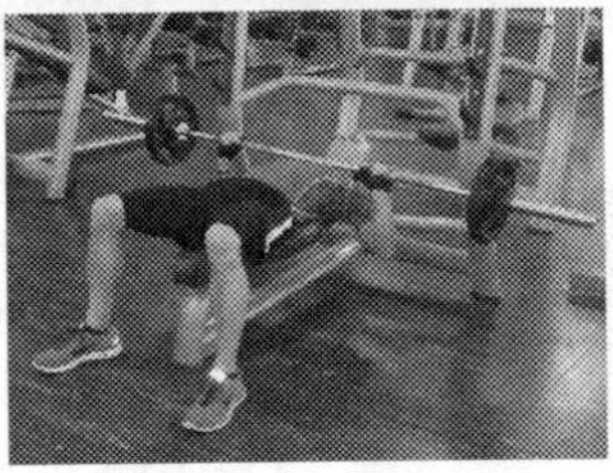 Most are familiar with this typical gym exercise and bench. It is one of the most intimidating exercises for many people, especially women. Obviously, it shouldn't be. The diagram shows good form including when you are bringing the bar down to your chest your elbows should only reach about 90 degrees (maybe a shade more) before your press the bar back up. An important consideration is that if you're trying to get healthy you don't need a lot of weight on the bar. The bar itself is typically 45 pounds with no plates on it whatsoever. Guess what ladies that's enough to start with. You may think it looks silly. It looks silly for a guy to do that (although I did). As a fat bastard with bitch tits doing an exercise that is meant to help tighten/strengthen your chest 45 pounds was more than enough for me when I started. I don't have my exact sheets with me anymore but I don't think I ever even got close to my own body weight that is a typical measure of bench strength. Again, I wasn't trying to build muscle as opposed to getting lean and mean.

Incline DB press Chest	Upper	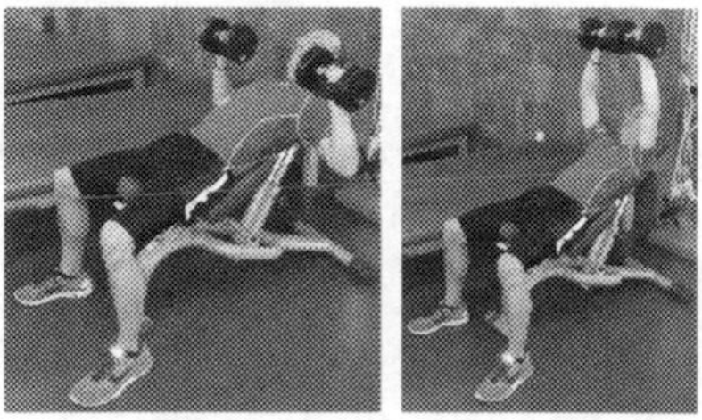 This is another good exercise to be done with a moderate amount of weight. Notice the arms come from a 90 degree bend or slightly more to straight up over your head. If you're using steel or iron dumbbells do not "clink" them at the top. If their rubber or plastic feel free to "clink" away.
Inverted Rows	Upper	Described on previous pages. I think I mentioned previously how much I hated these. Yeah, they suck but as with everything that's how they pay off.
Gravitron Pull Ups Wide/Back	Upper	Described on previous pages.
Gravitron Dips Chest	Upper	Described on previous pages.
Push-ups Chest	Upper	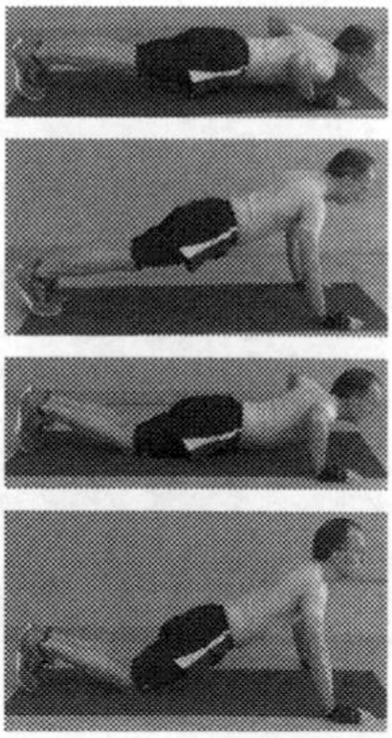 There are two forms of the classic pushups. They are sometimes referred to as men's pushups versus women's pushups. You'll be glad to know that this sexist position is completely crap. Fellow fatties... If you can only do the pushups with your knees on the ground than this is the way you should do them until you can do them on your toes like the picture on the top

Nautilus Lower Back	Upper	Described on previous pages.
Rolling Planks	Core	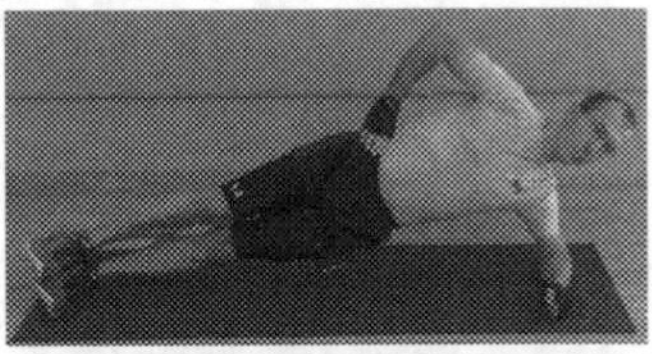 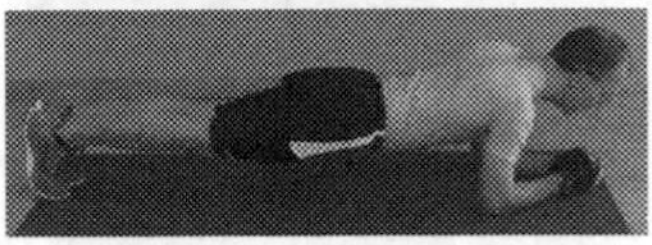 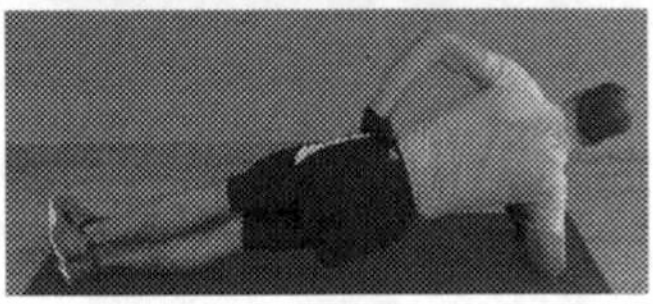 There are two forms of planks pictured above. They are, from top to bottom, the left sided plank, the classic plank and the right side or lateral plank. The plank pictured on the bottom is specifically, the "right sided" plank. Notice that for the side planks the feet are positions on top of one another. All pictures should show however that the back is PERFECTLY straight/flat (that is, like a plank or wooden board). This is important in this exercise because if the hips sag at any time during this exercise you can injure your lower back. When I first started doing these I had a difficult time holding the regular/classic plank for 30 seconds. I didn't even have the balance as a fattie to try the side planks. "Rolling Planks" is a combination exercise that starts on one side, say a left plank for 30 seconds and then, after 30 seconds, rolls over the regular plank and after another 30 seconds rolls into a right sided plank for a total 90 seconds. No rest in between the 3 sets of 30 seconds but you may rest after the 90 seconds. No more than half the time (45 seconds) before doing another set. Do 3 sets. I have had hundreds of people (hopefully thousands by publication time) ask me the single

		best exercise to tighten their abs and help get rid of their beer bellies or guts. THIS IS IT. No weights, no special equipment, no trainer or spotter needed. No matter your level of fitness this exercise is difficult for many to hold more than two minutes per position although it's a fun contest to try with friends. A special derivation on these planks is to do them with your feet elevated on a bench. This increases the work on both your shoulders and your core. Have fun, do them with EVERY workout. You'll hate them in the beginning and when you see that gut start to disappear (thanks to your cardio) and tighten up you'll love them. By the way gentlemen, if you can do a plank for 5 minutes straight it will pay off in the bedroom, trust me!
Crunches with Medicine Ball	Core	Described on previous pages.
Medicine Ball Twists	Core	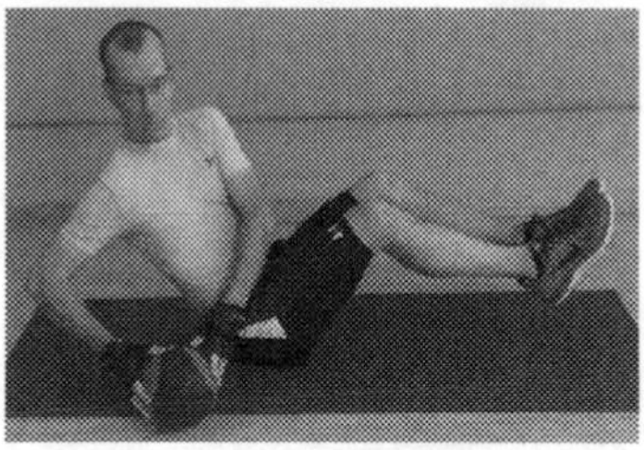 Another classic but a great one. Hated them forever, learned to love them. The trick that you will have to master with this exercise is keeping your feet off the ground without falling backwards. Also, when bringing the ball to each side make sure your twisting from the hips and touching the medicine ball to the floor. Use a middle weight ball. Maybe 10 to 12 pounds for the men and at least a 6 or 8 pounds for the women. Do 15 reps x 3 sets.

Leg Lifts	Core	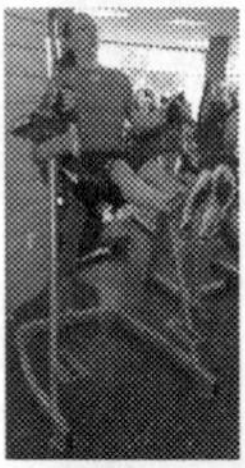 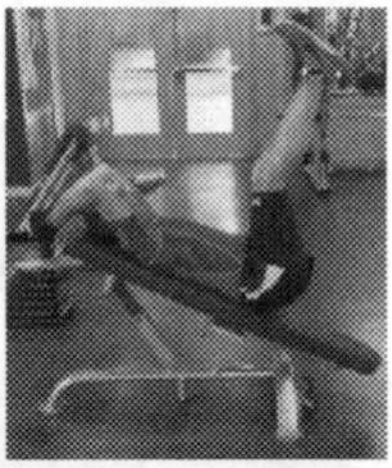 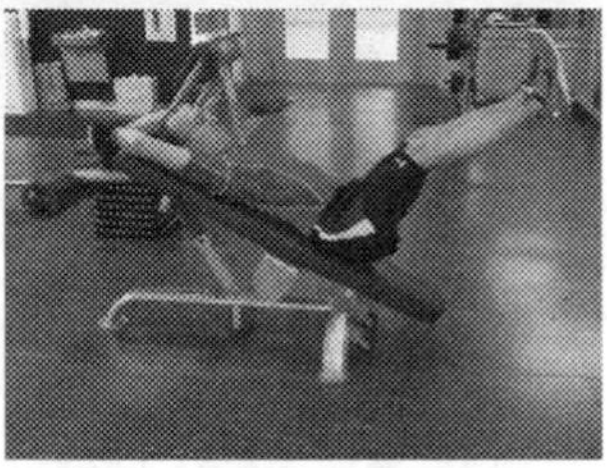 These pictures represent two different types of leg lifts. My routines started with the ones on the top right with my head at the elevated end I would grab the bar or the bench behind me and raise my legs to be 90 degrees to my body as the lower picture shows. Work that core baby. Abs and lower back. The picture on the top left is another piece of equipment at the gym that looks intimidating. I can testify personally that this one is difficult until you've mastered the ones on the right. The leg lifts on the top left are probably harder than those on the top right but both are accomplishing the same effect. A difficult addition to the ones on the top right (which can be done on either side but I've seen done when you're laying) is to attached the ankle sandbags to your feet so you have an extra 2.5 – 5 pounds attached to each ankle before you attempt to raise them straight up. Ow, my abs hurt and tense up just thinking about it. Yay, abs!
Walking lunges	Lower	Described on previous pages.
Leg Extension (Quad)	Lower	Described on previous pages.
RDL Romanian Dead Lift	Lower	Described on previous pages.

Standing Calf Machine Can be done on a Leg Press machine as shown if the above machine doesn't exist at your gym	Lower	There are many different ways to do this exercise. The benefit of using the machine at the gym is that you can vary the amount of weight and build your calves as well as stretching the muscles of the lower legs including the Achilles. Another important note about the picture is that the person in the picture is going from the tip toe position to the point where his feet are at a 45 degree angle with the heels pointed downward and the toes pointed upward.
one arm DB press Shoulder	Upper	Described on previous pages.
Shoulder Press 2 holes showing	Upper	Described on previous pages.
Shrugs (Traps)	Upper	Described on previous pages.
DB side laterals Shoulder	Upper	Described on previous pages.
Triceps (Skullcrusher)	*Tricep*	Described on previous pages.
Preacher DB	*Biceps*	Described on previous pages.
Tri PushDown Vbar	*Tricep*	Described on previous pages.
Bicep Zottman	*Biceps*	Described on previous pages.
One arm DB ext _Tricep	*Tricep*	Described on previous pages.
Biceps Cable Curls	*Biceps*	Described on previous pages.
Oblique ball toss	*Core*	Described on previous pages.
Torso Rotations	*Core*	Described on previous pages.

Superman's	Core	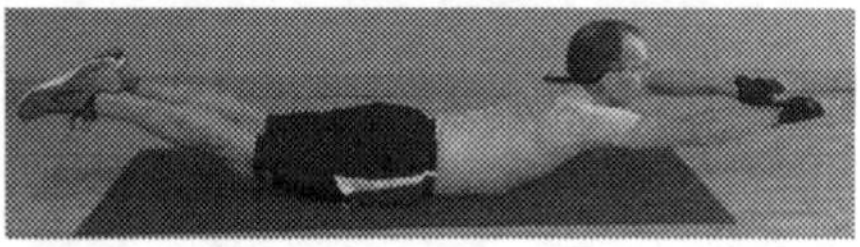 Why do these look way easier than they really are? I consider these almost as good as the planks and to some extent they are the exact opposite of the planks. Your object is to lie on your belly and raise your legs and arms like you are Superman and you are flying. Similar to the planks you should attempt to hold them for anywhere from 30 – 120 seconds with an equal amount of rest in between.

Since this is the "show me" chapter, I'm also going to reference the diet plan I previously mentioned. I spoke earlier in great detail about the number game I played with my dietician (i.e. the calorie Nazi), which she made me into as well. No, my Jewish friends, she didn't really make me a Nazi. Come on, you know me and my politics. The Nazi's were WAY too liberal for me. Again, if you don't know me personally or my sense of humor go hang around with people who have been firefighters, cops, or former military to get a clue about not taking yourself too seriously. You should be WAY more offended by your obesity than any possible word that comes out of my mouth or this book.

I spoke about how I started with a 3,000 calorie per day diet (including all the alcohol). I talked about how I scaled this down to 1,500 – 1,800 per day. One of the things I didn't mention earlier but will now is how little 1,500 calories per day is when you're used to eating TWICE that many. There's a yin and yang to this statement however. I do most things to the extreme. If I commit to something I'm "all in" as they say in poker. So, when Mary Ellen my RD said 1,500 – 1,800 I said, "OK, 1,500 calories it is." This amount of calories was difficult to accept; however, in retrospect, I am amazed at how much I was able to accomplish with so little calories. This dynamic was twofold. I had cut out the alcohol (all wasted, empty calories, with so much damned sugar converted directly to fat) and I had increased the basics including vegetables, and I even started using multi vitamins. The multi-vitamins I used were over-the-counter brands at first and then eventually getting into very specific vitamin routines that I'll talk about later. The second half of the dynamic above was that I was so FAT that the energy for my workouts was using my stored fat for energy as much as the more healthy food I was now taking into my body. What I found after a few weeks (about 8 – 10) was that my weight loss had reached a plateau and I stopped losing weight. When I went back to Mary Ellen and showed her my food log she picked right up on it and said something every fattie naturally loves to hear. "You're not eating enough." "What, how is this possible? You said 1,500 – 1,800 and I'm eating 1,500 per day." She explained that my body had adjusted to the amount of exercise I was doing every week and the reduced amount of calories I was consuming, so I actually moved my body into starvation mode and it was now conserving body fat.

Cool! I bumped up my calories to 1,800 and even allowed myself to go over on the weekends. Like magic my weight loss started a downward trend again and the additional calories gave me even more energy to do my daily exercise routines. Over the next several months, I continued to occasionally plateau, but with direction from Mary Ellen I was ramping up my calories at the same time from 1,800 to 2,100 to 2,300 to 2,600 to 2,800. Holy shit, I'm consuming almost as many calories at the peak of my weight loss as I was when I was eating like a pig. EXCEPT, now, it's 2,800 healthy calories (for the most part). After I continued to smash through one weight loss goal after the next, I became my own expert at dealing with the calories in my diet and how it affected my workouts and routines. After achieving my desired and maximum weight loss (85 pounds down from my original 235 pounds); I was at a place where I had reduced my calories from my max of 2,800 per day down to 2,700, and then down to 2,600, and then 2,200; and eventually back down to the 2,000 +/- where a normal healthy adult male should be. However, I am such a guru at the caloric intake of my body now I can adjust my caloric intake over a given week and add a few pounds or subtract a few at will when I know I have certain events coming up. That is, as an intermediate to advanced runner I know that I have to "carb load" and "bulk up" a little before a longer race (10K to half marathon) so the week or so before a race I'll allow myself to add two – five pounds because I know the extra "fat" and energy will be used during my race and I can use the next week to slim back to my goal weight. I have a digital scale in my bathroom and when I step on it I can tell you within 1/2-pound how much I weigh without even looking at the scale. When you have that sense of control over your diet and your own body, you will understand why you're reading this book and why you're altering your lifestyle to achieve the nirvana of healthy living.

Before I show some of my diet spreadsheets from the last few years, I said I would mention my vitamin routine. My vitamin regimen developed slowly from the time I started eating right until my two PTs kicked me in the head (not literally although it may have been needed) and said, "What do you mean you're not taking vitamins?" So, with their advice and Mary Ellen's, I started taking an over-the-counter brand name men's multi-vitamin. I'm not going to advertise their brand here, but I will go as far as saying I could get them at the company store I was working for at the time. At the time, I was a consultant, owned my own company (DAB Enterprises, LLC) and worked for Wyeth Pharmaceuticals in Malvern, PA. I'll let you figure out which multi-vitamin I was taking. Besides the multi-vitamin, I was also taking a fish oil supplement (two per day). I took all three "pills" in the morning with my morning water that also often contained the name brand vitamin C enhancement as well as an Airborne® tablet. I was addicted to overdosing on vitamin C as well as the multi-vitamin. As Mary Ellen told me it would have been very difficult for me to take too many vitamins based on my healthy diet and great exercise routine because whatever the body didn't need it would eliminate in the urine anyway. As always, the professionals were correct.

My vitamin regiment grew as my diet changed and my running and eventual competitive running increased. My vitamin need became very focused on enhancing my cardiac output and efficiency and continues to be the same to this day. I still take my vitamins every morning with a full 16 ounces of water (oftentimes with my same old vitamin C enhancement powder – even though I know at this point I don't need it). I've refined my vitamins to the type you can buy at the specialty vitamin stores (again – unless they're going to pay me I'm not going to name drop them into my book) but I do have a regular store I go to although if I run out and I have to pick up the more generic ones like fish oil or cinnamon, I still grab those at my local pharmacy (Walgreens, CVS, Target, Walmart, etc...). Yeah, cinnamon – regulates glucose and in my case is a positive mood stabilizer. Take one per day. My multi-vitamin requires two per day and they smell HORRIBLE, but they have EVERYTHING you could possibly need in a day. Work with your vitamin store expert to find the right multi for you. I prefer the type with the Energy Activated boost since I'm taking them in the morning (also the type with no iron – important for men unless you don't get enough iron). I mentioned fish oil already. Don't go cheap and belch up fishy breath all day. Go with a reputable brand that puts a drop of orange flavor in them and preferably find the largest milligrams you can (I use 720) so I only have to take the one per day. Potassium citrate (two per day) – show me a runner who doesn't need potassium supplements and I'll show you a runner eating bananas like a monkey cause you'd have to in order to equal just two little potassium caplets. Glucosamine/Chondroitin (750/600 mgs) – one per day at triple strength helps promote joint flexibility. Again, as a runner or anyone that does cardio, I believe this is a must do.

In the cardiac arena I take two vitamins that I consider almost more important than the rest combined. They're a little controversial because for every study you find on them that says they don't have the positive effects they claim, you can find other studies that say the opposite. I believe from my consumption of them that they are working for me. Try them for six weeks and then go without them for six weeks and determine for yourself if they have any impact. I take one of each, a 400 mg of CoQ10 (or 200 mg of Ubiquinol) and 300 mg of Alpha-Lipoic Acid. I believe that in cooperation with my running they are a partial reason why my cardiac efficiency has increased by over 12 percent in the last two years. All of these vitamins should be discussed with your doctor first, as I'm not one and I know what's worked for me. I know what I'm allergic to and what works for me. For instance, I got my father to take the Glucosamine/Chondroitin at one point to help with his joints. It would have worked if he hadn't developed a shellfish allergy in his 80s. He ate shrimp on occasion his whole life, but developed an allergy to shellfish in his mid- 80s. That sucked for him. Glucosamine/Chondroitin contains shellfish. It sucked more when he took the Glucosamine/Chondroitin and almost had an anaphylactic reaction. Funny that one of the many pharmaceutical companies I worked for during my extensive IT career was the company who sold EpiPen Auto-Injector®. I've been allergic to penicillin, sulfa, bee stings and South American fruit (mango, guava, and papaya) amongst other things most of my life, so I know what to avoid but as you change your diet it's not a bad idea to include your RD or doctor in those changes.

OK, onto the food logs. I'm going to show representative examples from different periods of my journey. I will attempt to show logs from ***April 2011, August 2011, October 2011, March 2012, June 2012, October 2012, and April of 2013***. I hope through these examples you will see some of the fads I mentioned above and trends in total calories I traversed during my journey. I will discuss some of the nuances of each below each one.

Food Logs

Meals for Week	Monday 4/4/2011	Calories	Tuesday 4/5/2011	Calories	Wednesday 4/6/2011	Calories	Thursday 4/7/2011	Calories	Friday 4/8/2011	Calories	Saturday 4/9/2011	Calories	Sunday 4/10/2011	Calories
Breakfast	Coffee + Slimfast	225	Coffee + Slimfast	205	Coffee + Slimfast	225	Coffee + Slimfast	225	Coffee + Slimfast	205	Coffee	150	Wrap+Egg+ Ital Saus+Cheese	**490**
Snack	Nutrigrain x2+ H2)w/ AB/EC	340	Nutrigrain	120	Nutrigrain	120	Nutrigrain	140			Starbucks Bfast Wraj	270	H2O+PP	30
Sub-Total Calories		**565**		**325**		**345**		**365**		**205**		**420**		**520**
Lunch														
Vegtable (1c)	Salad	30	Salad	30	Corn	140	Mixed	160	Broc	120				
Vegtable (1c)	O&V	168	O&V	168	A1	40	A1	20						
Starch (1/2c)	Cheese	45	Cheese	45			Rice	100	Rice	100	Blackberries	171	Iced Tea x2	120
Protein (6oz)	Steak	318	Steak	251	Chicken	280	Chicken	140	Chick Saus Apple	320	Strawberries	48	Slimfast	190
Snack	Apple	60	Apple	60	Apple	60	Apple	60	Apple+ H20w/AB/EC	90			Carrots	38
Sub-Total Calories		**621**		**554**		**520**		**480**		**630**		**219**		**348**
Dinner														
Vegtable (1c)	Carrots	105	Corn	140	Beets	140	Broc	120	Broc	100				
Vegtable (1c)									Rice	150				
Starch (1/2c)	Rice	100			Rice	100	Rice	100	Tilapia	210	Thai	668	PB&J	430
Protein (6oz)	Breaded Chick	340	Turkey Kilbasa+ Ital Saus	340	Chick Saus Sundried	280	Turkey Kilbasa+ Ital Saus	340	Soda	80			Sushi	387
Sub-Total Calories		**545**		**480**		**520**		**560**		**540**		**668**		**817**
Snack	Blackberry 1cup	98	GS Cookies (x15)	480	Strawberries+ GS Cookies (3) + H2O w/ PP	174	Strawberries+ H2O w/ PP	78	Girl Scoutingx10	320	Snack+ GS Cookies (x5)	480	GS Cookies (x5)	160
Sub-Total Calories		**98**		**480**		**174**		**78**		**320**		**480**		**160**
Cumulative Calories By Day		**1829**		**1839**		**1559**		**1483**		**1695**		**1787**		**1845**

April 2011

The first menu above – WOW, this is the first time I've looked back at it in a VERY long time. Let's see what I see that was a funny trend versus what I've since learned or changed. First, in relative terms I have to soak in the whole menu as this was the beginning of my journey, so I was slowly phasing myself out of shit eating into healthy choices. I mentioned my twice a week salad that has gone away as I now cannot tolerate that much "roughage" in my diet. I can't afford to be shitting my brains out any more. I know, disgusting right? If you've made it this far in the book I'm sure you can handle worse. Why? Because you're fat and if you've made it this far you've already made a commitment to yourself. You may not even realize it at this point, but you have. Good for you! You will have my support and if you continue to make the change, you will gain your biggest cheerleader – you! So, other trends from above. I was obviously still into the Turkey Kielbasa despite the ton of sodium, but if was fewer calories than much of the crap I was eating, so I took the hit on sodium. It was a fair trade at the time.

GS Cookies = Girl Scout Cookies. I see those under snack. HA! That makes me smile. I also noticed A1 which is the steak sauce. Yes, you must record EVERYTHING that goes into your body (except water – you can drink as much of that as you want). I notice apple as my snack. It's funny that I've since gotten out of that habit of eating apples; but that's because of other reasons that I will change again soon and probably go back to apples. Ah, I was still in NJ at this point so I see my typical Saturday meals were still eating out at the local Thai restaurant that I loved so much. Holy hell, how the hell did I only eat 1,483 calories on April 7th, 2011? I like that I was doing the Slim-Fast shakes as my morning replacement meal. I completely forgot about those, but they were an important part of my beginning phases. There are a lot of abbreviations in these spreadsheets. I'll try and hit most of them although as I continue to say throughout this book; this is what worked for me; these are not endorsements of these products or their manufacturers. If these people pay me for product placement, I'll say that but they haven't and suspect they won't because of the language of this book. It's not very politically correct and most people, especially corporate America, doesn't like that. I can tell from above that some of these vegetables were canned. I've since moved to microwave steamed veggies, but I could use some beets back in my diet so I may have to reconsider that again. I can see I still tried then as I do today to regulate the weekends without a lot of planning. I think that works better for me today than it did back then but it was a learning process. I'm almost excited to see what comes in the following menus.

Meals for Week	Monday 8/1/2011	Calories	Tuesday 8/2/2011	Calories	Wednesday 8/3/2011	Calories	Thursday 8/4/2011	Calories	Friday 8/5/2011	Calories	Saturday 8/6/2011	Calories	Sunday 8/7/2011	Calories
Breakfast	Slimfast+Coffee	195	Slimfast	190	Slimfast+Coffee	195	Slimfast+Tea	250	Slimfast+Coffee	190+5	Egg Wrap+ CB(x3)+Chese (x2)	415	Egg Wrap+ CB(x2)+Cheese	350
Snack	PBJ Wrap	200	PBJ Wrap	200	PBJ Wrap	200	PBJ Wrap	200	PBJ Wrap	200	PowerPack+G2+ QO Bar	165	Protien Shake	252
Sub-Total Calories		**395**		**390**		**395**		**450**		**200**		**580**		**602**
Lunch														
Vegtable (1c)	Salad	50	Garden	80	Peppers x2	60	Broc/Cali	60	Garden	80	PBJ	200		
Vegtable (1c)	Mush+pepper+ Cheese	155			H20+AB/EC	30							Nachos	345
Starch (1/2c)	O&V	167	Pastina (2 oz or 4Tbsp)	210	Pastina (2 oz or 4Tbsp)	210	Pastina (2 oz or 4Tbsp)	210	Pastina (2 oz or 4Tbsp)	210			Wine	300
Protein (6oz)	Steak	442	CS+CB	270	CB+CS	270	TK	315	IS+CS	330			Eggrolls (X1.5)	300
Snack	Walnuts+Apple	260	Fruit+Yogurt+ Walnuts+Apple	500	Fruit+Yogurt+ Apple	300	Fruit+Yogurt+ Apple+Health Snack Mix	423	Apple+Walnuts+ H2Ow/EC/AB	290			Thai Egg Rolls	150
Sub-Total Calories		**1074**		**1060**		**870**		**1008**		**910**		**200**		**1095**
Dinner														
Vegtable (1c)	Broc	60	Broc/Cali	60	Broc	60	Broc	60	Broc	60	Tilapia Filets+Sauce	336	Rice (2c)	480
Vegtable (1c)									Coffee+Almonds	105	Rice (1c)	240	Veg	30
Starch (1/2c)	Pastina (2 oz or 4Tbsp)	210	Pastina (2 oz or 4Tbsp)	210	Pastina (2 oz or 4Tbsp)	210	Pastina (2 oz or 4Tbsp)	210	Pastina (2 oz or 4Tbsp)	210	Shrimp (x6)+Soup	118	Soup	50
Protein (6oz)	IS+CB	340	1/2 TK+CS	287.5	IS+CS	330	IS+CB	340	1/2 TK+CS	287.5	Walnutsx2+Cherrios	520	Wine	100
Sub-Total Calories		**610**		**557.5**		**600**		**610**		**662.5**		**1214**		**660**
Snack	Protien Shake w/ Banana	247	Oatmeal x2+ Banana	345	Oatmeal x2+ Banana	365	Protien Shake w/ Banana+NutriGrain	467	White Wine+Oatmeal x2+Wine+Cherios	630	Wine	300		
Sub-Total Calories		**247**		**345**		**365**		**467**		**630**		**300**		**0**
Cumulative Calories By Day		**2326**		**2352.5**		**2230**		**2535**		**2402.5**		**2294**		**2357**

August 2011

Here we are only a few months after the last menu and I can see improvements in my nightly snacks. They've transitioned from Girl Scout Cookies to oatmeal (although I remember at this point this was still the Quaker Oats instant oatmeal that was yummy but had too much sugar). I eventually learned to use plain, rolled oats, and add some cinnamon and honey. I can also tell, big reveal, that this is after June 2011 when I "fell off the wagon" for good; but never let the wagon get too far ahead of me in case I needed to jump back on. Thankfully, by the grace of a Higher Power I have not had to jump back on but I am cognizant that it's always there. Pastina was a favorite starch of mine. This is also a good starch that's worth re-exploring in my current diet. I see apples and bananas, which are GREAT fruits. Bananas have become a thing of the past because they're so hard to keep from turning nasty down here in Florida or putting up with the fruit flies that come with them in the humidity here. I'm still on the Slim-Fast shake for breakfast kick. Wow, at least eight months in and that's still holding up. Impressive! Good job old fat, getting healthy, Dale. Probably the biggest holy shit is the shift from 1,500 calories up to an average of 2,300. At this point, I was working out so much that the body needed the extra fuel to do the workout, but was burning these extra calories and more. A few more abbreviations... PBJ = Peanut Butter and Jelly Wrap. PBJ wrap is a great breakfast snack around 10 a.m. I had two tablespoons of peanut butter (180 calories), two tablespoons of low sugar jelly (40 calories) and an 81 calorie low-carb wrap (8" shell). At the time, I was only using one tablespoon of peanut butter and a different type of wrap. The formula above is since I've found the right wraps to use. The low-carb wraps I found in the "ethnic" (Mexican) isle are perfect. IS = Italian Sausage. Yummy but loaded with sodium. As mentioned earlier, I have since moved away from the four-legged meats. CS = Chicken Sausage. As stated many times, it was a fad. It was delicious and low calorie. Sodium was insane as it's the classic "processed food". Everyone always tells you to not eat processed food. While the comment is true that's easier said than done when you're trying to ramp down from a life of gluttony. TK = Turkey Kielbasa. Better then a hot dog (not much from a sodium perspective but a bit healthier).

A friend who I was helping train recently wrote me an email and asked my advice on fuel (ergo the food she consumes). "I need to be more prepared, which I'm working on… for these early morning workouts." Here is my response/email to her relative to the running I was doing on that given day…

…REALLY funny you should say this about your fuel. Four a.m. came and went this morning but I was up at 5 a.m., so I got here, to the gym, by 5:30. I said, "Perfect, I'm in early so I'm going to do a 15K on the treadmill instead of my usual 10K"… Yeah, not so much. I got to mile 4.5 and said, "Wow, I'm only halfway to a 15K. I'm so screwed. No way I'm making it 9.3 miles, so I'll be happy with 6.2. I'll plan on doing 6.2 tomorrow morning."

So, to your point, as I'm at 4.5 miles, I'm thinking, why am I having issues? I look at the clock and I know my body; so as long as I have the time (I was early after all) I don't stress about speed. BUT, when the body says "nope, tank is close to empty," you have to listen to your body. Two things I screwed up on… If I knew I wanted to do nine miles this morning (before I woke up this morning) two things I should have ABSOLUTELY done (in my case – everyone is slightly different). I should NOT have had 1/2 glass (4 oz) of wine last night. Bad move No. 1. I can run a 10K on empty no problem. Bad move No. 2. I cannot run a 15K to a half marathon on empty. I needed to have had a bowl of oatmeal this morning, and I didn't want to do it because I'm also trying to slim down a pound or two before some upcoming speed work I have planned. It's all inter-related. I can cut calories and lose some weight, but if I do that I'm going to sacrifice endurance and distance. It's a simple formula. If you don't put fuel in the tank you're not going to go too far. A 1/2c of oatmeal with 1T of honey would have let me hit those last three miles. A banana and maybe a GU® packet would have done the same thing. BUT, the fact is, in my case I know what I can run on empty (you should figure out the same thing). After that you need 100 calories per four miles (very rough calculation) but basic enough for most people to handle.

You really have to play with it (and here's where it gets tough over email so bear with me). You are going to go through periods while you're running and trying to figure out what you should and should NOT eat pre-run or during run. You will have "gas" (from the top and bottom of your body). You will feel like you want to throw up. You will feel like you're going to "need a diaper." A very funny and honest coach laughed at me once and said "you haven't shit yourself during a run yet Dale? You're not a real runner yet." I can testify I'm not a real runner yet, but I've come VERY, VERY close to being a "real runner" more than a few times; so I can tell you this is what it takes to figure out your own personal, perfect formula for success. It will change as you lose weight, too. Right now you can rely more on your stored energy (that is, fat). As you lose weight and your endurance raises and your stored energy (excess weight) goes away you'll burn leaner fuel. Right now you're filling your tank with 87 (gasoline equivalent). I use 93. Your eventual goal is to burn 93. Mine is to burn jet fuel. Different goals but same end result. I hope that helps. We can certainly talk more about specific types of fuel you're thinking about. PBJ = GREAT, Bagels = GREAT. Fruit (pre run) = NOT great (without a diaper). GU® or other gel = necessary evil.

Meals for Week	Monday 10/3/2011	Calories	Tuesday 10/4/2011	Calories	Wednesday 10/5/2011	Calories	Thursday 10/6/2011	Calories	Friday 10/7/2011	Calories	Saturday 10/8/2011	Calories	Sunday 10/9/2011	Calories
Breakfast	Slimfast	190	Slimfast	190	Slimfast	190	Slimfast	190	Slimfast	190	Bagel Sammy	600	Pancakes/Syrup	510
Snack	Coffee+PBJ/Pita	305	Coffee+PBJ	315	Coffee+PBJ	315	Coffee+PBJ	315	Coffee+PBJ	315	QO Bar	90	Ham + G2	85
Sub-Total Calories		**495**		**505**		**505**		**505**		**505**		**690**		**595**
Lunch														
Vegtable (1c)	Salad	38							QO Bar	90			1/2 Turkey Hogie + Goo	380
Vegtable (1c)	Mush+ Cheese	75	Broc/Cali	60	Broc	60	Broc	60	Broc	60	Mii Grob	300	Wine	400
Starch (1/2c)	O&V	167	Rice	180	Rice	180	Rice	180	Rice	180	Thai Mussaman w/ Tofo	870	Bagel Sammy	645
Protein (6oz)	Steak	548	CB+IS	340	TB + A1	340	CB+IS	340	TK	280	Orange Chews	40	G2	45
Snack	Apple+Yogurt+ Fruit	300	Apple+Yogurt+ Fruit	300	Apple+Yogurt+ Fruit	300	Apple+Yogurt+ Fruit	300	Apple+Yogurt+ Fruit	300				
Sub-Total Calories		**1128**		**880**		**880**		**880**		**910**		**1210**		**1470**
Dinner														
Vegtable (1c)	Broc	60	Beans	60	Beans	60	Broc/Cali	60	Garden Medley	100	3 Cheese Ravs	400	Gnocci Dinner	548
Vegtable (1c)	Banana+QO Bar	195	Banana+NV Granola	285	Banana	105	Banana	105			Salad	153	Bread	350
Starch (1/2c)	Pita	80	Rice	180	Rice	180	Rice	180	Rice	180	Carrot Cake	350	Pasta Fagoli	360
Protein (6oz)	TK	280	CS x2	280	CS + IS	330	CS + CB	270	CB x 2 + A1	300	Iced Tea x3	30		
Sub-Total Calories		**615**		**805**		**675**		**615**		**580**		**933**		**1258**
Snack	Protein Shake+ Health Snack Mix	460	Protein Shake+ Health Snack Mix	548	Protein Shake + Oatmeal x2	617	Oatmeal x2 + Protein Shake + QO Bar	582	Oatmeal x2 + Cherios x2 + Pickled Veg	521				
Sub-Total Calories		**460**		**548**		**617**		**582**		**521**		**0**		**0**
Cumulative Calories By Day		**2698**		**2738**		**2677**		**2582**		**2516**		**2833**		**3323**

Holy crap! Still doing the Slim-Fast shakes for breakfast. I sincerely hope the makers of this product pay for some stuff eventually. I'll endorse, more vigorously, it for a nominal fee. But, in all seriousness, 190 calories was the perfect meal. They were yummy (especially the strawberry flavor) and quick, which were both important criteria at the time. I was also still doing Thai on Saturdays. I am a creature of habit for sure. I was allowing myself pasta on the weekends. Cool! Wow, how come I keep miss noticing the total calories until I finish writing up the menu: 3,323 calories. WOW! And 400 calories of wine is two 8-ounce glasses. I remember these nightly snack nights going over 500+ calories. Wow, this really helps put even my current menus into perspective because it really helps me reflect on how much time I was putting into my workouts and exercising. I was a true gym rat, but I was seeing the benefits and I was addicted to losing more weight. I'm telling you, you will be, too, and you should be. The results are worth the effort. At least I finally started to move to PBJs for breakfast. I see a healthy trend there that continues until this day.

Meals for Week	Monday 3/5/2012	Calories	Tuesday 3/6/2012	Calories	Wednesday 3/7/2012	Calories	Thursday 3/8/2012	Calories	Friday 3/9/2012	Calories	Saturday 3/10/2012	Calories	Sunday 3/11/2012	Calories
Breakfast	Real Oatmeal+Honey	210	Real Oatmeal+Honey	210	Real Oatmeal+Honey	210	Real Oatmeal+Honey	210	Real Oatmeal+Honey	210	Bagel Egg Sammy	485	Bagel Egg Sammy	440
Snack	N&J + Coffee	325	PB&J + Coffee	305	N&J + Coffee	325	PB&J + Coffee	305	N&J + Coffee	325	Real Oatmeal + Honey	210	Real Oatmeal + Honey	210
Sub-Total Calories		**535**		**515**		**535**		**515**		**535**		**695**		**650**
Lunch														
Vegtable (1c)	Salad	30	Salad	30	Broc	60	Broc/Cali	60	Garden	80	Pumpkin Seeds+ EnergyBar Crumbs	248	Hummus+Chips	177.5
Vegtable (1c)	Mushroom	15	156g Tomatoes	28.1	Salt Bagel w/ PB	530			Fruit	200	Wine	150	Popcorn	640
Starch (1/2c)	O&V + Cheese	193	O&V + Cheese	193	Rice	140	Wrap	110	Wrap	110	Energy Bar	250	Thai Soup	350
Protein (6oz)	Steak	300	Steak	345	Tofu	202.5	Tofu	202.5	CB (GF) + A1	150.0	Wine Pinot???	150.0	Mussaman Curry	600
Snack	Apple + Banana	165	Apple + Banana	165	Apple + Banana	165	Apple + Banana	165	Apple + Banana	165				
Sub-Total Calories		**703**		**761.1**		**1097.5**		**537.5**		**705**		**798**		**1767.5**
Dinner														
Vegtable (1c)	Fruit + Yogurt	240	Fruit + Yogurt	240	Fruit + Yogurt	240	Fruit + Yogurt	240	Fruit + Yogurt	240	Mozzarella Capresese	352		
Vegtable (1c)	Garden	80	Broc/Cali	60	Cali	60	Cali	60	Broc	60	Gnocchi (250/c)	500		
Starch (1/2c)	Rice	140	Rice	140	Rice	140	Rice	140	Rice	140	Sauce (1c)	362		
Protein (6oz)	Patty + A1	303.0	CB (lt) + A1	130.0	CB (GF) + A1	150.0	CB (lt) + A1	130.0	Patty + A1	303.0	Dessert+Bread+oil	504		
Sub-Total Calories		**763**		**570**		**590**		**570**		**743**		**1718**		**0**
Snack	Energy Bar + Sunflower Seeds	899	Hummas Wrap +Sunflower + Cliff	734	Banana + Cliff + Tea/Honey	390	Banana + Cliff + Tea/Honey	450	Pudding	208	Espresso	1		
Sub-Total Calories		**899**		**734**		**390**		**450**		**208**		**1**		**0**
Cumulative Calories By Day		**2900**		**2580.1**		**2612.5**		**2073**		**2191**		**3212**		**2417.5**

Finally moved away from Slim-Fast shakes to a "real breakfast" of oatmeal and PBJs or sometimes I would substitute Nutella for the peanut butter because the extra 20 calories for the same amount of Nutella was worth the tradeoff. I was still doing pasta on the weekends as well as Thai. I was still doing salads. That's interesting. A year into my program and I'm still doing salads twice a week including "with steak" on one of them. Average calories count is starting to drop now that I've reached my goal weight by this point in the process. It's still pretty high at 2,570 (average) but not as high as the previous period that was an average daily calorie count of 2,767. That 200 calorie difference was a big difference.

Meals for Week	Monday 6/18/2012	Calories	Tuesday 6/19/2012	Calories	Wednesday 6/20/2012	Calories	Thursday 6/21/2012	Calories	Friday 6/22/2012	Calories	Saturday 6/23/2012	Calories	Sunday 6/24/2012	Calories
Breakfast	Real Oatmeal+Honey	210	Real Oatmeal+Honey	210	Real Oatmeal+Honey	210	Real Oatmeal+Honey	210			pancakes+ syrup	465	egg wrap + Lentils	455
Snack	PB&J + Coffee	326	N&J + Coffee	346	PB&J + Coffee	326	N&J + Coffee	346	PB&J + Coffee	326			Energy bar	753
Sub-Total Calories		**536**		**556**		**536**		**556**		**326**		**465**		**1208**
Lunch														
Vegtable (1c)	Salad	20	Salad	20			Chia Water + cookie	220	Fruit + Yogurt	240	beer	190	Shrimp Burger	387
Vegtable (1c)	Mushroom	7	Mushroom	8	cookie	220	Beans	60	Mix	140	Mahi + Sauce	200	Lobster Tail	245
Starch (1/2c)	O&V + Cheese	193	O&V + Cheese	193	curry quinoa	196	lentils	120	lentils	120	FF + Conch Fritters	375	CousCous	365
Protein (8oz)	CB	197.1	CB	197.1	hummus wrap	210	TB + A1	380	hummus wrap	210	Wine	150	Apple	50
Snack	Apple	60	Apple	60	Apple	60	Apple	60	Apple	60	Wine	600		
Sub-Total Calories		**477.1**		**478**		**686**		**840**		**770**		**1515**		**1047**
Dinner														
Vegtable (1c)	Fruit + Yogurt	240	Fruit + Yogurt + Energy Bar	491	Fruit + Yogurt	240	Fruit + Yogurt	240	Fried Zuch	150	Crab	150		
Vegtable (1c)	Beans	60	Mix	140	Broc	50	Broc	50	Bread	350	Spinach	30		
Starch (1/2c)	lentils	120	curry quinoa	196	lentils	120	curry quinoa	196	Lobster Rav	1000	Orzo	180		
Protein (8oz)	TB + A1	380	Tofu	175	CB + A1	217.1	Tofu	175	Wine	300	Dessert	275		
Sub-Total Calories		**800**		**1002**		**627.1**		**661**		**1800**		**635**		**0**
Snack	Spaghetti + Wasabi	833	Energy Bar+ Pineapple+ Snacks	543	energy bar+ hemp+ wine	661	Energy Bar + Egg Wrap+	717.5						
Sub-Total Calories		**833**		**543**		**661**		**717.5**		**0**		**0**		**0**
Cumulative Calories By Day		**2646**		**2579**		**2510.1**		**2775**		**2896**		**2615**		**2255**

The initial June spreadsheet I used contained my birthday week, so there were a few things that were "misrepresentative" of my menus for this time period. The menu above more accurately reflects what I was going through at this point. The important point from above I realized is that this is one month after I moved from New Jersey to Florida. And relative to the previous period, I was still at approximately the same calorie consumption rate – somewhere between 2,500 and 2,600 per day average. Another important point from above is that I was bulk loading the end of the day (after or post dinner). Some of the lessons learned I can appreciate from this menu and pass along to the reader as "experimental." This was my first month in a new area of the country. And, while I LOVE, south Florida everything and everywhere takes adaptation and getting used to. So, I experimented. Never before this month will you see conch fritters on any of my menus. There was a phase I went through for a period of doing hummus wraps because while hummus is delicious and having it in a wrap was brutally simple to prepare, I was really eating it because I was so happy to be living so close to a Whole Foods grocery store; I was really taking advantage of the fresh ingredients and my new local shopping options that were not as prolific in New Jersey. Another thing that I can reflect on from above is my willingness to make my starches not be the same every day. I actually made half of the week as one type (lentils) and the other half the other type (quinoa). I need to get back into this to spice my menu these days because it's too easy to get wrapped up in "easy preparation," which leads to boring and that leads to diversion from the menu.

Note that the line above in the menu that mentions hemp is referring to the natural hemp seed. I have not done nor have I ever done cannabis. Almost all (not all) of my girlfriends wish that were not the case, but sadly it's true. I don't have anything really against it other than the smoking aspect, which I became hyper-sensitive to growing up as my mother smoked cigarettes like a chimney and I always hated the smell of the smoke; it drove me to really dislike anything smoking related. Of course, being brought up in an Italian family that statement is a bit of a contradiction because many of my uncles smoked nasty cigars. While I hated those smells worse than the cigarettes my mother smoked, the cigars became a memory of my youth. As I got older and eventually started playing golf in my 20s and 30s I would occasionally have a cigar while I was golfing. In retrospect, I NEVER liked them but I found the smoke was reminiscent of my childhood and the positive memories of my uncles and family gatherings. Thankfully, I never developed a "taste" for this disgusting hobby. If any of my readers enjoy cigars, I apologize but you will find that your exercising WILL be inhibited by your use of tobacco products (no matter its form). The stimulant the tobacco provides is not a body altering chemical you need if you would only exercise more. Anyway, that was a tangent from the menu, but it was one of those brain recollections being stimulated by the whole hemp conversation. Sorry about the distraction; back to the menu.

Meals for Week	Monday 10/1/2012	Calories	Tuesday 10/2/2012	Calories	Wednesday 10/3/2012	Calories	Thursday 10/4/2012	Calories	Friday 10/5/2012	Calories	Saturday 10/6/2012	Calories	Sunday 10/7/2012	Calories
Breakfast	egg sammy and fruit	330	Egg White Omlette + Cheese	295	Egg White Omlette + Cheese	295	Egg White Omlette + Cheese	295	Egg White Omlette + Cheese	295	Bagel Sammy	490	Egg Wrap	272
Snack	PB&J + Coffee	325	PB&J + Coffee	325	PB&J + Coffee	301	PB&J + Coffee	301	PB&J + Coffee	301	Gu x2 + Banana x2 + OJ	510	Pumpkin Bar+ Mocha Java	330
Sub-Total Calories		**655**		**620**		**596**		**596**		**596**		**1000**		**602**
Lunch														
Vegtable (1c)	Food at TycolS Days		bad	176			Coffee Mocha	70	Cookie	172	fallafel sammy	300	wine	300
Vegtable (1c)	chick bbq	200	Broc	50	Beans	60	Broc	50			fallafel balls	150	energy bar	250
Starch (1/2c)	pasta	400	Rice	180	Rice	180	Rice	180			yogurt	250		
Protein (6oz)			Tofu	350	CB	174	Tofu	350			wine	100		
Snack			Apple	60	Apple	60	Apple	60	Apple	60	pumpkin bar	130		
Sub-Total Calories		**600**		**816**		**474**		**710**		**232**		**930**		**550**
Dinner														
Vegtable (1c)	Fruit + Yogurt	240	Fruit + Yogurt	240	Fruit + Yogurt	240	Yogurt (Fruit Bad)	140	Fruit + Yogurt	240	Gnochii	228	fish taco	776
Vegtable (1c)	Beans	60	Broc	50	Broc	50	Wrap	81	Pasta	768	Sauce	175	Mushroom	150
Starch (1/2c)	Rice	180	Rice	180	Rice	180	Rice	180	Sauce + Cheese	235	Cous Cous / Quinoa	320	Pumpkin Bar	130
Protein (6oz)	TB	380	CB	174	TB	380	CB	174	Ultra	95	Ultra x2	190	Yogurt	450
Sub-Total Calories		**860**		**644**		**850**		**575**		**1338**		**913**		**1506**
Snack	Oatmeal;	210	G2 + Ice Cream	320	Oatmeal x2	420	GU+Bad	188	Snacks	240				
Sub-Total Calories		**210**		**320**		**420**		**188**		**240**		**0**		**0**
Cumulative Calories By Day		**2325**		**2400**		**2340**		**2069**		**2406**		**2843**		**2658**

October 2012

We're now getting closer and closer to the present day of my writing of this book; and I notice trends that have emerged and conformed to my rigorous schedule of the past. By the way, Sammy = sandwich. That is, the ability to know when to "let go" and trust yourself. That concept certainly started before this menu but in the increments that I'm including in this book it represents the first such proof of that concept. Another aspect of this menu that is CRITICAL is that in the month prior to this menu (September of 2012) is when I actually stopped eating all red meat (defined in my book as anything that, while it was alive, walked on four legs). While I've probably slipped up a little on this with the occasional breakfast sausage or piece of bacon since September of 2012, I can officially say "red meat" is no longer an element of my diet. There's good and bad to this philosophy, but mostly good. I say more on that challenge in a minute. Analyzing other aspects of this menu I see that the Monday lunch was spent at a company event where we were provided lunch at a company BBQ. Again, "let go and let God." That is, it's OK to "cheat," it's OK to go "off plan" or "off menu" once in a while. As long as you document (afterwards) honestly and accurately, you can account for the divergence either way. If you went to a company event and stuffed yourself on goodies and sweets, so be it. Document it and add up all the calories (or Google how many were in each yummy treat). You'll use the rest of the week to make it up.

I'm only going to recommend this once you have full control over your menu, your calories, and your ability to "let go" but "take inventory and when you were wrong promptly admitted it and corrected it without harming anyone else." That's a little 12-step humor built into the chapter for those obese people who are also addicts reading my book. Laugh at yourself, if you're reading this book than I hope/pray you are also conquering your other addictions or addictive personality traits. June of 2012 began to demonstrate my Friday night pasta night, which has preceded all of my Saturday morning long runs since I moved to Florida. The weekends still tend to be "all over the map" but that's OK as long as it's documented. I recently explained to someone that I can now shift my body weight by 5+/- pounds in any week depending on what I'm trying to accomplish. Do you understand how powerful that is to your mind? I want to add a few pounds during this particular period (between Wednesday and Friday) because I know I'm going to need the energy from the "fat" for Saturday morning (my typical long runs) and that I'm going to burn much of the excess off; and that will also keep my weight-loss cycle continuing into the following week where I'll lose the pounds again. Some weeks I choose to use the week to shed those few pounds so I can "lighten" the load for a fast 5K I'm trying to tackle. For the most part, this book is the "101" version of this Healthy Living lifestyles. There are more advanced books I can write (and may in the future) to talk about controlling you weight on an "as needed" basis, and adjusting based on workouts, events, and planning for "life." This is what happens when you're making plans for the future. Another note from above is that I went off and on throughout all of my menus on my fruit/yogurt consumption. I have really never nailed this aspect down, except to say that each is good and both together are better. I do, however, use this morning snack as a bit of calories playground. I may have mentioned previously that keeping bananas fresh in the Florida heat is no small challenge. I was doing apples every day and bought two slicer/core removers for home and work. Eventually, frankly, I got tired of apples because the mixed fruit was easier and "different."

Meals for Week	Monday 4/29/2013	Calories	Tuesday 4/30/2013	Calories	Wednesday 5/1/2013	Calories	Thursday 5/2/2013	Calories	Friday 5/3/2013	Calories	Saturday 5/4/2013	Calories	Sunday 5/5/2013	Calories
Breakfast	Egg White Omlette + Cheese	154	Egg White Omlette + Cheese	154	Egg White Omlette + Cheese	154	Egg White Omlette + Cheese	154	Egg White Omlette + Cheese	154	Oatmeal + Heed	310	DAB Bar	251
Snack	PB&J + Coffee	306	PB&J + Coffee	306	PB&J + Coffee	306	PB&J + Coffee	306	PB&J + Coffee	306	G2	130	Nut bar+Red Bull + Marshmello	490
Sub-Total Calories		**460**		**460**		**460**		**460**		**460**		**440**		**741**
Lunch														
Vegtable (1c)									dessert	125	tofu bacon wrap	300	Pita + Soy Cheese Egg + Espresso	241
Vegtable (1c)	Broc/Cali	60	Beans	60	Broc/Cali	60	Beans	60	rice panir	255	organic macaroons	250	Veggie Juicer	180
Starch (1/2c)	Rice	170	Rice	170	Rice	170	Rice	170	veg sauce	230				
Protein (6oz)	Tofu	175	CB	194	CB	194	TBx2 + A1	400	naan	300				
Snack	Yogurt	240	Yogurt	140	Yogurt	140	Yogurt	140			wine	150		
Sub-Total Calories		**645**		**564**		**564**		**770**		**910**		**700**		**421**
Dinner														
Vegtable (1c)	cookie	86	fro yo	450	cookies	350	cookie	175			mee grob	300	sea bass (52/oz)	840
Vegtable (1c)	Beans	60	Broc/Cali	60	Beans	60	Broc/Cali	60	cheese	60	salad/soup	150	beets	40
Starch (1/2c)	Rice	170	Rice	170	Rice	170	Rice	170	pasta + Sauce	875	red curry	790	tofu	141
Protein (6oz)	TBx2 + A1	400	CB	194	Tofu	175	CB	194			ice cream	100		
Sub-Total Calories		**716**		**874**		**755**		**599**		**935**		**1340**		**1021**
Snack	ultra x1 + Crunchy + Popcorn	445	ultra x2	190	egg wrap + ultra + pumpkin seeds	508	egg wrap+pumpkin seeds	332	ultra	190	Ultra	190	wine	400
Sub-Total Calories		**445**		**190**		**508**		**332**		**190**		**190**		**400**
Cumulative Calories By Day		**2266**		**2088**		**2287**		**2161**		**2495**		**2670**		**2583**

April 2013

This menu is only one month before I began writing this very chapter. The first thing that jumps off the page at me and needs to be addressed (because I'm not sure if I did earlier in my menu analysis) is that there is Michelob Ultra and wine represented on this menu as "snacks." First, there's no place else to put them, so they had to go somewhere; and as time went on I was less concerned about where food items were placed on the sheet and more particular that all food items be placed on the sheet. Second, many of my friends from the various programs I've been over my 12-step paths will question why I would allow myself to have alcohol anywhere in any diet plan, no less advertise it to a bunch of pigs who have little self-control. It is purely to demonstrate that we are all weak and we all have our vices. You are not Gandhi or Mother Teresa. There are few people in the history of this planet that are that pure. Admit it; acknowledge you failings and shortcomings and aspire to do and be better, but if you're going to diverge from the healthy menu plan for God's sake at least write it down.

Since June of 2012 I was also on a frozen yogurt kick so you'll often see FroYo listed as a snack and usually listed at 450 – 500 calories. I didn't eat that much frozen yogurt but all those yummy toppings that often accompany that frozen yogurt will get you every time. I'm a particular fan of wet walnuts, raspberry chocolate cups, peanut butter cups, and cinnamon sauce on my frozen yogurt. The frozen yogurt itself may only be 150 calories, but the other crap brings it up really quickly. Again, I'm not going to deny myself this treat, but I am going to document it.

Friday lunches also became a tradition with two of my work colleagues. One guy was Indian and the other British, so the three of us all loved Indian food/curry; so this became our weekly venting/working session where we'd solve the problems of the company, and then move on to world peace and conquering hunger. Ha! Anyway, if you were to look at every week you'd see this Friday pattern for a significant period of time and only changed if one or both of my colleagues (or I) weren't in on a particular Friday.

So, this was my plan, I know that chapter/section was almost 50 percent of the entire book, but I think that's the point. You wanted to know how I did it. Well, now you know. So, with that let's move on to talk about the results of this plan.

RESULTS

The final section of my book has been a long time in coming. I wasn't sure how it was supposed to end for the longest time. I got a ton of advice from everyone I spoke with about the subject. Should I end it by doing a marathon? Should I end it with pictures? Should I talk about all of the amazing things that have happened in my life since losing all the weight, and keeping it off for almost three years now? I should talk about all of these things and more. I will even give you a bit of the negative that comes with the incredible amount of positives. What you will also be happy to hear is that this chapter will not be the longest in the book. I truly hope it's the shortest because what will turn out to be a section or Chapter Five about the "how" I did it will surely be the longest portion of the book. This chapter was intended to be somewhat short and sweet. What I want you to get out of this chapter are the promises I will make you, if you choose to live a healthy lifestyle.

Let me start off in my usual fashion that I hope you've come to love by now. If not, to hell with you!

So, you fat bastard or fat cow as the case may be. You are or were a morbidly obese, pathetic, piece of crap. You have or are about to put that moniker behind you. You will be transformed over the next several months (or have been already) from Fat Ralph or Obese Martha to Skinny Ralph or Slim-n-Trim Martha. You are the one everyone at work says, "Oh my god, how did you do it? What's your secret?" You will proudly tell them that there is no secret. You either choose to be fat and disgusting or you choose to live healthy, but at the end of the day you choose the healthy route. It's based on your strong mind, willpower, faith, and belief in yourself. I certainly hope my book and my inspiration helped as well. As I've been trying to preach to you all along. If this fat bastard can do it, ANYONE can. I had no willpower, I was weak, the food, the lifestyle, and the booze had a death grip on my life and it was choking skinny Dale to death. Through a searching and fearless inventory of myself and a situation where I was forced (through a series of life events) to focus on myself (whether I wanted to or not) showed me the light and the path. Some people have asked if I replaced one type of "aholic" with another. Well, if I've become a workout-aholic or health-aholic than seriously? Go screw yourself. If you think that's bad, I have news for you. There are way worse routes I could have gone and I can guarantee a few of them would have had me dead by now.

So, let's start with the positives. This is really the reason you made it this far in the book. Let's talk about all of the amazing and awesome things that have changed in my life since I choose to live a healthy lifestyle. I will break it down into physical (the most obvious), psychological/emotional, and metaphysical/spiritual.

Self Image

Let's get physical. Duh, did you see the cover of the book? For God's sake man, I'm a stud. OK, maybe I'm still the bastard child of George Clooney and David Letterman, but compared to Fat Dale, Skinny Dale is the man I've been hiding for 41 years. I'm so happy to see him finally emerge from the folds of stinking fat that this is the first positive physical trait I will list because it may sound cliché, but it's the truest thing I will write in this chapter. The No. 1 positive is that this transformation has given me the gift of sight. What are you talking about Dale? You were blind? Your eyesight got better? You don't need glasses anymore? It's way better than those! When I look in the mirror I actually make eye contact with the person in the reflection. I smile and say, "Nice, where the hell have you been? God, I needed you over the last 20 years." The reflection usually says, "I've been here all along fatso, why'd you take so long to look me in the eye – because you were shamed, disgusted, embarrassed, suppressing emotions? Well, are you done with that shit now?" Yes, yes, I am! I can confidently say I can finally look at myself in the mirror and be happy with what I see. This is the No. 1 physical accomplishment I've made beside the actual weight loss.

I will talk a little bit more about the physical because while it's not me to gloat over this type of success, I cannot deny that it's an integral part of my success at living healthy. When I first started losing the weight (as the title implies) at an average of 10 pounds per month, my PT at the time Chris G was adamant about the weight-training I was doing. Thank god he pushed me and was there for me, always designing programs that met my need and propelled me to the next level. The muscular definition that took place in my arms, my chest, my abs, my back and even my lower half like my glutes, hams, calves, and quads is remarkable. I hated doing planks in the beginning. I still hate doing inverted pull-ups, but damn it they are great exercises. I actually look forward to planks now and have become an evangelist for what I believe is the No. 1 exercise that all fatties with a belly should be doing. You want to shape your abs? Do a perfect plank, do it on the side, do it on a ball, do it elevated, but do them and do them often. All of the definition and work that Chris helped me do on my legs made me a stronger runner and allowed me to continue that hobby as a passion, and improve at it with fewer injuries than I otherwise would have incurred. I rarely work on legs anymore as running takes care of them now for me, but I still do an occasional circuit/cross-training class that hits multiple muscle groups during a workout.

Far be it from me to leave this out from my final chapter. I've laid out so much of my personal life and embarrassing stories that why should I stop now? I mentioned earlier in the book about one particular part of a man's body that actually grows when you lose weight. Again, I can attest with a total weight loss of about 81 - 85 pounds (I maintain weight between 150-155) there is a certain appendage that actually becomes significantly larger thanks the increased muscle of your lower abs; and the plethora of testosterone and lack of estrogen now pumping thorough your body. Sorry ladies, there is not a similar effect on the female side although I've been told that the female sex drive does spike quite a bit due to the same hormonal adjustment that your bodies are making. Seems like a pretty good reason to me for you to consider losing all the weight. However, I know the ladies will focus more on my ramblings related to the psychological/emotional positives that I'll speak to more in a few paragraphs. Trust me, male or female, these are worth the work as well.

"Strength" (physical, mental, emotional, spiritual) / Endurance

Let me mention another physical trait of getting healthy. Endurance in everything you do. I will keep this paragraph focused on physical endurance. How many of you fatties get winded going up one flight of stairs? How many of you smoke or even if you've now quit smoking, previously smoked for years, get winded doing the simplest activities? How many would like to coach or be a more active part of your kid's sports teams, instead of just being the fat mom/dad being the cheerleader in the stands? Physical endurance for me translates to some of the following activities that as Fat Dale were laborious at best and downright distasteful/abhorred at worst. I've often ended up (not on purpose just the case) living on the third floor or higher of my apartment buildings. Steps sucked! Now they are easy and sometimes I look at them as a mini-workout that motivates me to stay healthy. The simple act of carrying groceries from your car to the house/kitchen has actually become another fun/humorous activity to see if I can do everything in one trip. This is a dual strength objective/goal, but it really combines both strength and endurance (especially if you live in an apartment or more than a few dozen feet from where you park your car to your home). Endurance has helped me become a far better lover to my partners. I mentioned earlier in the book that I'm a flaming heterosexual, but that makes no difference to the abilities you will develop by getting healthy. Straight, gay or bi-sexual, you will appreciate the benefits (as will your partner) of being able to maintain a "plank" position for minutes at a clip. See, there's even exercise you can incorporate into your lovemaking (just try not to actually think about working out while you're with your partner – takes away from "the moment"). God forbid you start counting while you're doing it. One, 2, 3, 4, 2, 2, 3, 4, 3, 2, 3, 4… could get you to meet the Lorena Bobbitt in your significant other. Don't say I didn't warn you.

I mentioned definition of muscles earlier, but I left out the obvious strength component. I mentioned it above in a simple task like carrying groceries but again, this applies to everything you do in life. Whether you're a blue-collar worker in which case it could actually make you more efficient at your job, netting you bigger rewards. You'll see that things that used to be difficult at work and at home are now easier because of your new physical strength. Carrying luggage is easier. Picking up heavy boxes is easier. Picking up your spouse, your kids, objects around the house; they will all become easier.

Let's talk Psychological/Emotional positives now. I've already alluded to, if not specifically said, that the ability to look in the mirror and actually look myself in the eye and FINALLY be satisfied with the body/shell that's looking back at me is an amazing feeling. I look at the definition in my chest, the nice cap of the biceps, the V of my waist as it heads downwards and tonality of my quads and calves leaves me bewildered by how much a human body can change when it's motivated to do so. When I see the image in the mirror is allows me to walk around inside and out without a shirt with complete confidence. There's no way anyone could look at me and make any type of negative comment about the physical appearance of anything from my neck to my waist. Wow, that's a long way since "bitch tits." I notice not just the definition in my forearms when I'm running or exercising, but the actual veins and how when my pulse is racing or my blood pressure is pumping hard that these veins are raised/stick up showing. It reminds me how healthy my body has become on multiple levels. Perfect levels are related to every blood test you can run. Perfect blend of proteins, fats, carbs, and essential vitamins/minerals is coursing through my veins and I appreciate the healthy choices I've made in the last 3+ years.

Having a positive self image has positively affected every area of my life from work to personal. When you have confidence in your appearance, and in your ability to deal with almost any situation, you can much more easily overcome obstacles. You can bust through roadblocks that others will, so easily, throw in your way.

I talked about the physical endurance that I've gained and how every woman I've been with has always been appreciative of that level of physical endurance. Well, along the same lines under the topic of psychological, I have mental endurance that can now transcend what I thought I couldn't do. Whether I need endurance for sexual reasons or just to deal with my boss at work, I have more mental capabilities to that with my new exterior shell now. I know what it's taken me to shape my body and how long the process was. It constantly reminds me that nothing worthwhile comes easily or quickly and dealing with life situations can be psychologically facilitated, if you have confidence in other areas of your life.

Let me think for a second and I'll encourage you to do the same thing... What areas of your life could be improved if you had an increased self-confidence about yourself, your body, your image, your physical abilities, or your psychological prowess? Let me think about the things that have been facilitated by a positive self image... My ability to deal with the opposite sex is near the top. My confidence at work is definitely number two. In my world, these are really the top two things I need help with every day. In your case, maybe it's a renewed self-confidence that drives you to improve your golf game, your relationship with your spouse, your relationship with family members; maybe it inspires you to help others accomplish a similar goal to what you were able to accomplish. The possibilities to improve your life and lifestyle can be truly endless, if you have a positive self-image and no longer need to put yourself down because you are too fat.

Relationships

I mentioned relationships above. Let me speak to how some have improved, some have gotten worse, and some are just different. There are both positives and negatives to these relationships. Again, let me stay positive for now and focus on how my relationships have improved as a result of me following a healthy lifestyle... Having a ton of self-confidence reinforced a behavior that I had begun a few years earlier. When I began my charge of "brutal, unadulterated honesty" the first time I did it as a defense mechanism to hide behind all of my emotional baggage of fatness. It was a joke. I was being honest, but it came out more "mean" than honest. Oh, it was honest, but maybe too honest. Well, having the confidence of healthy living and a positive self image enabled the same behavior to occur without the meanness behind the tonality in my voice. I was able to be honest with my girlfriend(s), my co-workers, and a very important contingent, the people who have worked for me as my direct reports. I have been a better manager and leader since I lost the weight than I ever imagined I could be, and I'm only getting better as time goes on. How did my personal relationships with girlfriend(s) get better, especially if I use that noun in the plural? If your honesty is so great Dale, why don't you have a "permanent" girlfriend? The process most kids go through early on in their life of trying to find the "one" is the process; I didn't start until I became skinny Dale and found that while dating I could be completely honest and expect the same from my "partner in crime." Unfortunately, most people I end up dating have a problem with unfiltered honesty. Based on the experiences I've had in my life, including the salty ones, I've included in these pages and the dozens and dozens more where I've only skimmed the surface. I feel ultimate and total honesty is the path for me.

My direct reports in my career of Information Technology have benefited from absolute honesty because I can tell them areas for development without any bias towards anything other than what's in the best interest of their career. I had a fantastic mentor of mine tell me once, "Dale, if everyone that reports to me gets to be a CIO (Chief Information Officer) before I do than

I know I'll have done a great job." I wasn't sure if I could ever be that humble when he made that statement to me 13 years ago. Skinny Dale can now reflect on it, understand it, and process it. There have been moments where some of the people who have worked for me in the past have superseded my own career; and I know it had a lot to do with my encouragement and guidance at the time when we worked together. I was happy for them and glad they did well and even felt proud that I had contributed to their success; but there was a piece of me that was still jealous of their success. Skinny Dale "gets it." I can now, not only appreciate it, but accept it, and be truly happy for those people. So, if they're reading this now, they should know I am truly humbled by their amazing efforts; and it was a privilege to work side-by-side with you at one point in our careers.

Let me talk about relationships with friends. This is a tough one to be positive about, but I will do my damnedest. The reason it's so difficult is because a majority, not all, of my relationships since the age of 20+/- have been based on Fat Dale and his perspective. I think when I look back over the last 20 years of friendships/acquaintances I've had (outside of work and immediate family), I can break them up into three distinct categories. These three groups may or may not reflect your situation as well. I look at these three distinct groups as the enablers, the bystanders, and the inner circle. How does Skinny Dale look at these groups and respectively say that they represented 90 percent, 9 percent, and 1 percent of all the relationships I've had in the last 20 – 22 years. Skinny Dale has perspective on my relationships. Skinny Dale has a new found wisdom that comes with age and experience. Not the experience of living day-to-day life, but the experiences that try a person's inner core and test their true metal. Will they crack under the pressure? My journey to healthy living and the road that I had been down previously took me to the depths of the darkest places in my soul/essence/spirit. I know and have seen uncontrolled rage, human depravity, human cruelty, and savage behavior in others and in myself. This has allowed me to be honest with everything within me.

About 90 percent of the people that I've known for the last 22 years enabled the behaviors that made Dale fat. It's not their fault. There is no blame here. They were merely objects in my space that were reacting to my own actions and my own reactions. Newton's first law is the perfect analogy. One of the many positives I learned in AA is that you MUST separate yourself from your triggers. What are the things in you that trigger your fat behavior? Is it people, places, things, events, times, seasons, or other areas? In my case I had to physically move from Collegeville, PA to Hillsborough, NJ to get away from a majority of my enablers. The reason this paragraph is still based on the positive is because I say, as I mentioned earlier, I have no ill will towards ANY of these enablers (people, places, or things). I merely had to separate myself from these enabling and triggering events to be able to focus on myself and getting healthy for the two years I lived in New Jersey. I do not wish to "divorce" myself from these people, but the distance that I've put in between me and them (both physical and mental) is on purpose and for my own health.

The bystanders are a smaller percentage (9 percent). These are the people, places, and things that were merely "there" as I cruised through my journey as fat Dale. What I am sorry for at this point in my reflection is the "people" that were bystanders during these 20 years. Some of them may have even reached a hand out to help along the way, but I honestly don't remember. If you offered and I looked away or refused, I apologize and I thank you for your offer. My life had to take the path it took. There was no other way. Again, I see this as positive because I have the ability to look back and identify certain individuals and places who were bystanders who may have even been hurt by Fat Dale. I am remorseful and I can tell you that as I said earlier in this book, "karma's only a bitch if you are." Well, trust me bystanders, karma caught up with Dale. It bitch slapped me good. So if you were a bystander and tried to help by never enabling my wicked, evil, fat behaviors then you are a truly amazing and wonderful person. You were not the reason Fat Dale was who he was. I hope that someday these people and places can be a part of my life again. Many of them still are (the people) but I look forward to returning to certain places that only knew Fat Dale. The people who were in the bystander group I would consider friends. I hope, when this book actually comes out, that people don't ask me if they were in this group unless they really want to know where they stood. I think I can say, like so many other things in life, if you have to ask, you're probably not in the group.

The inner circle is easily 1 percent of the people I have known in the last 22 years. I can assuredly count on one hand the people who have gotten to know EVERY corner of Fat Dale; and a few of these inner circle members have started to get to know Skinny Dale. They see the dichotomy in the before and after. They can appreciate where I came from, where I went to, and where I'm going.

With a quick review of what I've said above I realized that I didn't say anything about family. I know many of my readers are probably wondering this as they have close relationships with their families. I can most easily put my family into the same three buckets I've mentioned above. I can with assured certainty tell you that no one in my family is within the inner circle, so that means they fall into one of the other two categories. I know I'm being vague about one specific subject in particular. I think I can address it quite simply. Where the hell do your parents fit into this Dale? They must have been in these three groups somewhere, how have you dealt with that? Suffice it to say, my relationship with my parents (who are still alive as of the writing of this book) were and are absolutely a huge part of my journey of epiphanies. Group? Well, obviously they fall into the enabler category. I think I can honestly say, without remorse, that they are probably the King and Queen of the Land of the Enablers. But, again, as I said above, I cannot hold ill will towards them for that. As my 12-step brothers and sisters know, "they did their best and if they knew better they would have done better." At least that's what we tell ourselves in meetings. I believe that statement.

The only contradiction from above is that while I have distanced myself, both physically and psychologically, from most of my enablers, why then did I move to Florida where my parents are living (at the time of this book writing and where they've been for almost 25 years)? Despite what I told many of my employers, getting to Florida was personal (for Dale) WAY more than any other influence. Sure, did the line, "I moved here to be close to my aging and elderly parents who are not long for this planet" sound like a great line in an interview? Sure it did. And it was/is true. However, the emphasis I put on that statement may have been a little hyped. Why would I want to move closer and become more involved with the King/Queen of Enablement? To truly understand and surmount my issues as Fat Dale (that were clearly based in my childhood and associated behaviors), I have to understand that which truly corrupted me in the first place. That probably sounds like a horrible statement to say that my parents "corrupted" me. It's not meant to be mean or ill willed but it's a fact that I cannot escape. Their drinking, their frequent and unfettered use or corporal punishment (both physical and mental/verbal abuse) and their response to a traumatic event that occurred within our family around the time of my 16th birthday were the bedrock that allowed Fat Dale to build upon and "fester" with shitty self- destructive behaviors for over 20 years. I can only hope that this book will help other fatties break through that wall before they waste as much time as I did. Or, even if it's been longer for them, at least they may at least know peace at some point in their lives.

Let me shift gears for a minute and speak to the less tangible benefits I've received in other areas of my psyche. This is a unique area for many that have known me. For those that don't know me as well (most of you) this will probably seem like an obvious point or two, and you'll probably wonder why it's not more prolific through the book. I will NOT let this turn into a soapbox. Those close to me know how easy it is for me to get on a soapbox about certain subjects and religious viewpoints is definitely one of them. I view religion much as I do many of the other areas of our American freedom. I believe we have inalienable rights to choose many things about the way we live our lives and conduct ourselves. I've said earlier that I believe in the "Golden Rule" and I believe it seems to be somewhat consistent in most religions. I've mentioned I believe in a Higher Power but am not sure, at any level, what that means, nor do I believe I'm supposed to. What's the result of Skinny Dale on these spiritual and metaphysical matters? I can certainly say that's it had an impact. I don't know if I classify it as positive or negative, but a change nonetheless. Personally, I believe that the concepts of karma, yin and yang, and a higher power have certainly grown within me during the last few years. No, my Christian born again friends and family, you will not be seeing me in church any time soon. I said they've grown but considering the depths they've reached, they're still at a five out of 100. I went from being raised Catholic to having no beliefs/faith to getting confirmed in college to going back to having no faith to a brief stint with atheism and landing squarely on "we are not the smartest thing in this universe and our existence here is more than just pulling ourselves from the primordial ooze."

Much beyond that profound acknowledgement I will not make. ☺ I will tell you that my belief in something greater than myself has increased. So, what does that mean Dale? Do you pray? Who are you thankful to when you do well in a race? If you were to die today would your "soul" go to heaven? If you participate in 12-step programs that are spiritual based, you must believe in God. Anyone who makes that last statement has never been in a 12-step program, but let me pull back the curtain for you… All 12-step participants come to believe in a power greater then themselves and whom some choose to call God. So let me answer your questions in the honesty you've come to expect from me. Do I pray? Yes. Who do you pray to? Because my life has only ever known Catholicism as the only organized religious group I've ever belonged, I use some of the basics from that religion as how I pray. Am I praying to Jesus Christ, the Saints, the Virgin Mary, etc…? Ah, no. Am I praying to a guy in a long white beard sitting on a cloud looking down over these ants we call six billion people? Maybe. Who am I thankful to when a race goes well? That's easy. I'm thankful to my coaches, my training, and myself.

Any "God" that has time to look over my race or the baseball, football, soccer, or other stupid human "sport" and guide it's outcome is one pathetic God, and the people who believe he's influencing the outcome of the Super Bowl really should be chlorinated from the human gene pool. If I were to die today would my "soul" go to heaven? I have no doubt there is an essence inside each human body. I spent over 15 years in the Emergency Medical and Fire Services. I have seen my share of dead people and a number of them have died in front of me while I was working on them (some clinically, some biologically). Based on my personal experience, I think I can say that there is something that leaves the body when this weak and watery physical shell we exist in shuts down. I don't refer to it as a soul. To me, it's more of an essence. People think of a "soul" going somewhere (to heaven, nirvana, etc…). I truly believe this essence disperses into the atmosphere. It is this essence within me that I draw on to motivate me to continue my training, my healthy living, and my new outlook on life. I hope that you can draw your essence in whatever form you believe to get healthy and stop being a fat burden on this planet. I respect and encourage you to believe it whatever form of a Higher Power you have to believe in to motivate yourself to do cardio, lift weights, play a sport, or just stop being the lazy fat bastard you are today. A summation of this point is that within the last year of my healthy living, I have begun to end everything I speak to with the word "peace." I am, in no way, referring to the hippy two fingers V salute. I am referring to a state of being and living. Be at peace with yourself. Be well, be calm and be peaceful.

I will end this portion of "My Results" with my wrap-up statement on the positive emotional and psychological results and where I am as of today; and where you can be as a result of changing from your evil, fat ways to a new lifestyle. At the end of each day, I need to be happy with myself and the last two years have put me closer to that goal that the previous 41 years. I hope and "pray" anyone who reads this can do the same. That is, try to be happy with yourself. You can do this by losing weight and getting in shape. I promise you that you will have a new outlook on yourself and life, if you can follow the advice and pattern I've set. If I can do it, you can do it! Now get out there and do it.

I've talked about success on many levels throughout this book. I think a success that many of us can relate to is the ability to control your own eating habits and weight as a matter of choice. If I decide on any particular week to add a few pounds for a week, I can choose to scale it down the next week properly. If I decide that tonight I want a FroYo after I go to see a movie where I had two beers and a bag of popcorn, I can do that because I know what it translates to in exercise and less calories the following day(s). The major point here is: I'm in control, not the food, not my addictions, not my demons, not "Fat Dale"... Me, I'm in charge and I can have whatever I want to eat. Can you think of a sweeter definition of success for a fat slob?

My personal life goals have even been easier by modeling them after my running/healthy goals. For many, that may sound like an odd statement. What I want to get out of this life is analogous to my running efforts because when I started "running" I was morbidly obese and what I called running was actually a moderately paced walk by my current standards. Three years later, that original pace that I was "jogging" is now my cool down walk after I've almost doubled the speed of that original "jog." Three years later I've entered my first full marathon after completing 25 other races of various distances from one mile to a few half marathons (13.1 miles). My personal goals of professional, personal, and mental/emotional success are put in perspective because similar to my weight problem, it took me 20+ years to fuck it up, what makes me think I can fix anything overnight? I can't, nor can you. It's a dumb cliché but it's painfully true that life is a marathon not a sprint. Similar to training for a marathon, you cannot simply go from no exercise to running a marathon without severely injuring yourself or worse. You often hear runners talking about enjoying the scenery along our paths. Again, too many (including me) never understood that. How can you concentrate on anything other than where your next breath is coming from? As you become healthier and a better runner you begin to understand this concept. Some of the pictures below are along my various routes that I run these days in Florida.

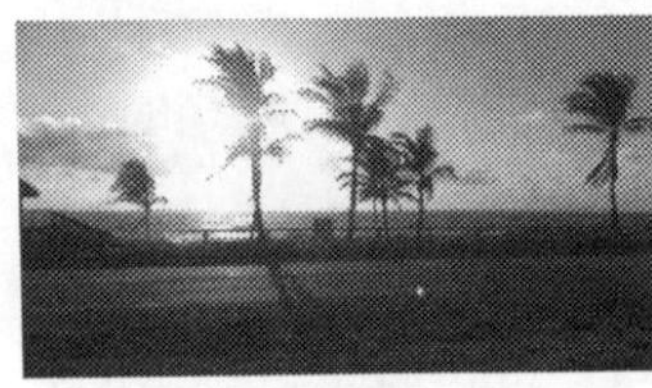

Early morning run along A1A in Boca Raton. Probably about 6:30 a.m. and I'm about an hour (or 6ish miles into the run). Every time a group of runners goes past this particular break in the trees, where you can look out at the Atlantic Ocean and see the sun backfilling the image of palm trees and waves crashing onto the beach, we remember why we're out here "torturing ourselves." It's for these moments, however fleeting.

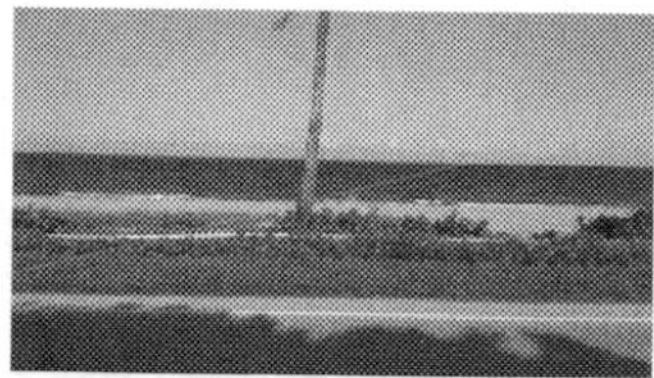

This is an after a run along the same stretch of A1A in Deerfield Beach (where I lived for a while in Florida). Gentle waves slowly rolling onto the beach.

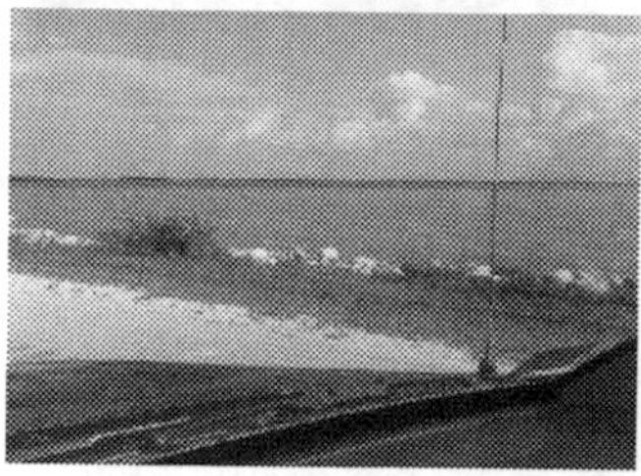

I took this picture out my windshield on the way back from a half marathon in Key Largo, Florida. As I was driving up Route 1 from the Keys to my home in Deerfield Beach, I noticed how clear the water was and that it was literally, only about 20 feet from the car on both sides of the road. The thought of driving in the middle of the Atlantic Ocean was humbling; but what gave me the chills was the fact that I had just run this stretch of road the day before in the race. I ran 6.55 miles with this scenery each way (that's 13.1 or a half marathon).

So, the moral of the above learning experience is that you will succeed at every life goal you set your mind to. You must dedicate unwavering support to achieve your mission to get healthy. Just like losing the weight, there are no secret formulas, there's no magic bullet, there's no "quick fix." It takes hard work, time, sweat, blood, and more than a few tears.

My original epiphany occurred on 1/1/11 in Key West, Florida. There have only been three New Year's eves since then, but I have endeavored to use each one to try and set some goals for the upcoming year not as resolutions (who can or really keeps those anyway). These are personal commitments to me. I am fully accountable to no one but myself. Each time I set these goals, I try to make them achievable within the year.

So what's next? Not just from an epiphany standpoint; not just from a personal development standpoint; where do I go from here? The dual-edge sword of achieving this much personal/health success is that I now want to share it with almost everyone I meet. This has translated into many thoughts over the last couple of years, such as telling Corporate America to go screw itself, go get my personal training certification, use my "success" from Corporate American to buy or open a gym in some awesome location like the Florida Keys. I could simultaneously get my life coach certification, market my DAB Energy Bars (more about those in a moment), and even potentially become a motivational speaker on getting other fat bodies like me to turn their lives around.

I can't believe this is the first time I'm speaking about my DAB Energy Bars. Part of my running program included experimenting with the dozens of products out there to keep yourself hydrated and carb loaded while you're running long distance. As a result, I've tried every type of energy bar, protein bar, and gel there is to try. Well, honestly, that's a lie because there are hundreds and I guarantee I haven't tried them all, but I've certainly tried. I was tired of trying everything from sawdust held together with agave to some gel that was good for the first 0.5 seconds it hit your tongue and then suddenly your body said to itself "oh, this isn't going to sit well in 20 minutes." Always listen to your body. Eventually, when I was reading an article in Runner's World, I ran across a recipe for making your own "health bars." It really sounded good and easy to make and since I fancy myself a decent cook, I figured I'd give it a try. I played with the recipe for a couple of months until I found what worked best; and even though no cooking of the bars is required, I do put the seeds into the oven to allow their natural oils to come out before mixing them in with the other ingredients. I will not give away the secret formula in case it turns out to be a hit, but I will tell you the same thing I put on the package. This energy bar contains the perfect blend of the four seeds known as the energy seeds of the modern runner. They are 100 percent natural, organic, and vegetarian! They are awesome cold (from the fridge) but are equally as good (just sticky) at room temperature. I encourage fellow athletes to have a bar before their exercise or after as a quick pick me up. I believe, personally, they are more beneficial before exercise because of the amazing properties of the seeds contained in the bar, especially the chia seed. Approximate calories are 251. Contents of the bars include: Granola w/ hemp, dried cranberries, almonds, chia, pumpkins eed, sunflower seed, low-calorie maple syrup, honey, margarine, cinnamon and vanilla extract. Keep refrigerated until consumption.

Let me talk about one of the ugly parts of exercising and getting healthy. I will remember to preface this brief chapter with I am not a doctor, although I occasionally have told a woman differently while I was at a bar. For the record, I am not a doctor of any kind (at least not yet). I want to reference injuries. I can only speak to what I've heard, seen, and encountered. When you move from just getting healthy to really becoming an athlete, injuries are more like "battle scars" and signs of accomplishments than negative points to be feared and stressed about. I've said, a few times throughout this book, that whatever form of cardio exercise you're doing, you must enjoy it so that you can shed the pounds and keep them off. For me, it happens to be running. In the world of runner athletes we often encounter other disciplined athletes like tri-athletes who complete triathlons (duh). A triathlon is a combination race where you typically swim, bike, and run (usually in that order). They have various distances from "sprints" to full Ironman's.

I was recently coaching a 0 – 5K program at our local running store and as we were sitting around stretching one day after a run one of the student runners asked, "how do I know if I'm overtraining." All of the coaches, including me, laughed as I answered her with a question, "Have you injured yourself yet?" She replied, "No" in a confident and proud tone. "Well then, you're not training hard enough." Injury is a part of training is like an alcoholic that says, relapse is part of recovery. Any athlete will tell you that the statement while sometimes true is an oxymoron. If you are ramping up your mileage from nothing to be able to run a 5K your body is going to go through changes as it adapts to the new demands you are putting on it. If you are a seasoned 5K runner as I was for the first 18 months of my getting skinny journey, and then you suddenly have this crazy idea that you want to run a half marathon your body will go through additional changes. These "additional changes" often involve some sorts of aches, pains, or other more serious injuries.

These injuries can be the most basic shin splints to more serious muscle strains or even worse tendon tears. I know I've said it previously about running but there is a foolish notion that if you want to start exercising you can find that old pair of sneakers in the back of your closet, throw on some cotton t-shirt and shorts and start jogging. Well, if that's what gets you out the door and into the habit then so be it; but be forewarned that if you are truly going to change your lifestyle to live healthier than you will soon find that having good and proper gear is VERY important to proper exercise. This is especially true to prevent or minimize injuries. I have personally had most of my issues initially with shin splints, then later lower back pain, and then eventually shoulder pain (right side); and most recently a fairly decent injury to my Achilles tendon that has been mending (while I continue to run on it) for over 9 months. Trust me, I'm tending to it with braces and special nighttime socks, but there is a reason that there are athletic stores that sell every kind of gear you can imagine. You think it looks silly until the first time your calf muscles tighten up to the point where your legs literally just give out and you fall to the ground in pain like someone just shot you. Athletes and people getting healthy become experienced with injuries. They become acquainted with a whole new field of medicine, which they probably never knew existed while they were fat. They learn to appreciate the holistic approach of massage and its importance in the relaxation of muscles and lactic acid release from those same muscles.

Let me also mention one of the negative areas of spending all this time getting healthy. It's an area that I could not have imagined; but I've learned so much about it in the last couple of years. Once I figured out the issue, it became apparent to me that while I couldn't do anything about it, at least I understood the issue. This reduced my anger on the subject. I started off this book talking about how 80 percent of the American public is fat. I vowed to myself that if I were able to get healthy/skinny I'd write a book about it and if it helps just one person, then I will have achieved my goal; the karma forces of the universe will reward me. Let's do another math problem for a minute. If I help one out of 350,000,000 Americans to conquer their battle over their individual obesity, I have helped exactly 0.00000029 percent of the population. In my book, that's a good job. What it means mathematically is that we healthy/skinny people are still in the minority (the 20 percenter's). Guess what being a minority means? That's right. As a skinny/healthy person, I can point to specific situations where I have been "discriminated" against because I didn't fit in with the norm. This even includes within the four walls of corporate America. As I can attest through my own screw ups; if you are a healthy/in shape guy or woman, do not go into an interview with a fat woman or fat guy and boast about your "extracurricular" activities like the gym, the road race, the Ironman, the triathlon, the tennis match, racquetball game, pickup basketball at the park, or even the golf round you just had (no matter how close to par you shot); you will most likely NOT get the job no matter how qualified you are. As of today, obesity is not a criteria that you can discriminate against, so there is also no such thing as "reverse discrimination" when it comes to not hiring healthy candidates. Same applies for women. If you're healthy and in shape the person across the desk will be intimidated by the number of yoga, Pilates, cross fit, Zumba, and 5Ks you do. Try not to make your potential business colleague uncomfortable with you too early. If, after you get the job, you can slowly convince them to change their sedentary ways, than great. The other funny part is that this can work both ways. You may notice that you are in a customer service role of some type and have made the conscious choice to get healthy/skinny and take care of yourself. If you, like me, are the boss or in that customer facing role, what is the FIRST thing that comes to your mind when an obese candidate or customer comes to you. "Oh, their lazy," "come on dude, if I can do it anyone can," "yuck, how disgusting, take care of yourself brother/sister"... Together we will slowly reverse this trend but like training for the marathon, it will not be quick or easy. It'll take time and more energy than we think we have. As I can attest, it's a good fight to fight.

One other negative I mentioned in the beginning of the book was about when I first went to a plastic surgeon to discuss my options. I said one of the comments he made to me ..."take half of what you'd spend on me, go pay a personal trainer, and come back and see me in six months, and I'll take off the excess skin for you and you'll be happier." Let me be frank with you that loose skin is not just ugly but... OK, it's just ugly. This is a little bit of a Catch 22 in that obviously you had to lose the excessive amount of weight in the first place to have this problem. The second Catch 22 is that if you followed my plan above or another personal trainer's plan, most people will not be able to tell you have an excessive skin problem. But, you will, and you'll quickly find out the ugliness of this issue. The number one way to fix the problem is to grow significant muscle to compensate for the skin that is excessive. Many people believe the skin will retract. That's only true for younger people and it also depends on how obese you were when you started. If all of your excessive skin (as is the case with me) is around your abdominal section, than surgery may be your only option. Tight abs does get you the consummate six-pack abs, but if there's extra skin around your belly that won't go away; you'll never see the six-pack, only the case the six-pack came in. In my particular case when I'm standing up straight (or vertical) you can't really tell I have excessive skin, unless you notice the stretch marks around the sides of my belly. However, when I'm in the prone (face down) position and especially if I'm with a significant other is when I really notice my issue. I have recently gone back (now that I live in Florida) to get a quote from a local plastic surgeon on removing the skin. It's not cheap (i.e. over $10,000) and not covered (since it's cosmetic) by most (certainly not my) insurance. There is no easy answer that I've come up with for this challenge, but I'd still rather be healthy/skinny with excessive skin than the fat bastard I was for most of my life.

The last topic I'm going to address in my book is a topic that I didn't consider much until I started helping others begin the process of losing weight. I actually heard from many people who were always trying to get to the end faster than they had any right to, "Dale, this all makes sense but once I get to my goal how do I MAINTAIN it? I've never been able to keep it off. You should write a book on maintenance." If you've paid any attention throughout this book, you'll know and understand why I finish this book similar to way I started it. That is, ANGER. I get so angry when people ask me this question about, "How do I keep it off?" "How do I maintain?" Did you just read a couple hundred pages of my life story and pay no attention? This is NOT a damn quick fix. This took me three years to conquer and like all addictions it'll be a lifelong process. Maintenance? You MORON, there is no such thing as maintenance. You're not "maintaining" anything. You're living your life like you've chosen to live it. That's not maintenance, that's a choice. You've made a choice to CHANGE YOUR LIFE. You've made the right choice. You've made the correct choice. You have done it, you've worked hard, changed your perspective on food (that is, fuel for the engine), and you've changed your attitude on exercise and incorporated into your lifestyle. You've CHOSEN! There's NOTHING to MAINTAIN! You're just living you NEW life. AWESOME! GREAT JOB! KUDOS! Now, live your life. No need to maintain shit. Just live. You've learned that with exercise and diet you can lose five pounds in a week without much effort at all. Once you've used my motivation and your own and obtained the weight-loss goal, you've learned how to live not how to maintain. Just set a weight trigger. Say your weight goal was 160 (if you're a guy) or 130 (if you're a woman). A guy would say that if he hits 165 (or alternatively 155) he needs to pay closer attention to calories in versus calories out. A woman may have a three pound trigger. When you've reached your trigger point, pull it and fix it. Will you continue to track your calories in and/or out on a spreadsheet for the foreseeable future like you're favorite author (me)? As of the writing of this book, I will have almost 250 spreadsheets and I can tell you on any given day in the last three years what I had to eat on any particular day for breakfast, lunch, dinner, or any of my snacks during the day. This includes holidays, vacations, weekends, or even "party" nights. It becomes a routine that you're more comfortable maintaining because you've seen the results of keeping track of your lifestyle and the benefits it provides. You've found that just when you think you've got it conquered and you stop "tracking calories" you start putting tonnage back on and you can't figure it out... I just had it, how did I lose it. Remember, I talked about our body's natural tendency to follow the route of least resistance. Maintain the discipline and you'll be fine.

So, that's it. You've made it. You came in with some notions about how I was going to help you lose your fatness. Did I meet your expectations? Were you able to accomplish your goals or are you at least on your way? The obese version of you will always be in your mind, but the skinny healthy version that you are so proud of… the version that you can finally look into the mirror and acknowledge, is the new and improved version of you. It's the version of you that you've rebooted and developed a new set of rules by which to live, work, and play. You have done what few people have the motivation to do. If you've taken any of my advice relative to a 12-step program, I would now encourage you to take my "Everything Your Mother Told You to Do," 12th step. Bring the message of healthy living and a healthy lifestyle to others who are fat, obese, morbidly obese or just plain disgusting. Confront them with the honest, ugly truth. Walk right up to them with your new skinny body and tell them they're a disgusting mess. They know it and you know it. You can say to them, "Dale said if he could do it, I could do it; and now that I've done it I'm telling you that you too CAN do it." It's possible, it's probable and it's necessary. So, put down the book, get motivated by another former fat bastard and make it happen. I cannot wait to hear your success stories.

APPENDIX A - MARATHON TRAINING...

I mentioned briefly in the last chapter that after 2.5 years of living a healthy lifestyle, I decided to be influenced by a friend to do something I never had a desire to do: Run a marathon. She said, and this was before the horrible bombing at the Boston Marathon, "I want to qualify for Boston next year. Will you train with me to help me?" That was around February of 2013. I thought about it for weeks because I knew what investment this would require. We researched races all over the US. We found two in Pennsylvania (east side of the state and one on the west side). We choose the west side and began training. We had different coaches and mentors, so we had different approaches for training. Both training approaches were valid. Her training format was to follow an overall program for tri-athletes because she was also training for many triathlons over the course of our training. My coach's philosophy was shaped by her Olympic qualifying time in 1992. "If you want to run long you have to train long." I believe in this philosophy; and while there are as many philosophies as there are coaches (including one that claims the longest run you will ever do is 15 miles before your marathon), I believe, for me, the right program was the one I succeeded with.

My coach's program was a four-month program. Our marathon was in September of 2013, so I started training long before the middle of May that was the official program kickoff. I had confidentially trained for and run half marathons, but this was a whole new level of commitment. There's nothing too confidential about a (half or full) marathon training plans so you should be able to Google many including some from Runner's World magazine and Marathon Guide.com. Before you begin this training plan you should be able to confidently run at least a 10K. What I learned about myself over the course of the six months while I trained for this marathon were as amazing as the weight loss I'd undertaken to get to this point. My friend (a 51-year-old female) wanted to qualify for Boston in 2014. Her qualifying time would have been anything less than four hours. I had no expectations for my first marathon, but I knew what time I could run a half marathon in, so I could estimate my time for a full. Sub four hours seemed like a good goal. There's probably a whole chapter or book I could write on my training for this marathon, but now that I'm writing this paragraph it almost seems like a distant memory. It would be almost anticlimactic. It's not really. It was a fundamental mile marker in my journey. Continuously ramping up my mileage from 25 – 30 – 40 – 50 – 60 miles in a week was an amazing feat. Amazing dedication that I never thought I could muster. Going from my normal weekend "long runs" of 10 miles to 15, 18, 20, 22, 24. Oh my God, I'm really going to do this. Am I crazy? Oh my God, I'm in so much pain. My nagging Achilles became a chronic pain that I've held onto to this day, nine months later. Go to a doctor they say. OK, so I can hear them tell me to stop running for two – three weeks to let it heal. Yeah, you don't know runners, do you doc? Sure, could I do elliptical or biking like I talk about in this book to stay cardio fit? Sure, I could, but that's not the point. Running has become the addiction. Running has become the lifestyle.

A couple of months before the marathon, my training partner fell off her bike during a transition phase in a triathlon she was competing in. She injured her ankle badly but again, like all stubborn runners continued to train and run on it for several weeks. About one month before the marathon her coach and she decided that running the full marathon would cause too much damage to her already hurt ankle. It was OK for her to run the half marathon at the same event, but not the full. She knew, with her injury that sub four hours was out of reach. A few weeks before the marathon, she decided to downgrade from the full to the half. I was personally deflated because I felt I started down this road because of her and her goal. Her goal had now become my goal. You learn when training for a marathon that injuries can and will happen. You learn that many people who start training for a full will not finish their training and may never actually get to the race. While I was disappointed, I knew that my partner's decision was not unusual. It helped me transition from helping a friend meet her goal to accomplishing the goal for myself, not just someone else. At the end of the day, come race time, this was the right mindset for me.

We still traveled to the race together and even stayed in the same hotel room. We had the traditional pasta dinner the night before and even met my original coach (KK) and his wife in Erie, Pennsylvania. He was also intending to qualify for Boston 2014. For me (and my coach who is the same age as me) it would require a 3:15 time. In my case this wasn't realistic. In his case, I wasn't sure how much, not if, he would beat that time by. September 15, 2013 came and we were in Erie, Pennsylvania for the Erie Presque Isle Marathon (and half marathon). So, why exactly would we train in Florida (during the summer) to run a 26.2 mile race that was 1,500 miles away from our home? Because, after living a healthy lifestyle for 2.5 years, and then taking six months to train for a goal that was for all intent a fantasy for 40+ years, it was only appropriate that it would require me to fly into my hometown (Buffalo, NY) and drive the 90 miles down to Erie, PA to compete in this race. And, after 3 hours, 53 minutes, and 51 seconds after the gun went off, I crossed the finish line in a burst of speed over the last 0.2 miles that I certainly did not expect in the last two miles before that. I had accomplished my goal; our goal; **MY** goal. It was the perfect culmination of 2.5 years of training, living healthy, and becoming the new me.

The weeks and months that followed that amazing accomplishment were challenging as it seemed like this was the ultimate goal, how could I continue with my own advice, set the next goal and get moving? After weeks of contemplation, I finally decided that while this was an amazing accomplishment (and I knew I didn't have a desire to commit to this level of training again, any time soon), I decided to re-focus on shorter distances and faster times. By how much could I PR a half marathon? Could I ever get to a 21 minute 5K (or less)? These were the new goals I decided to focus on. Oh, and I wanted to re-dedicate myself to trying to develop relationships and working certain 12-step programs around those issues. So much to do, sounds confusing. I know. New Year's is coming… How about another trip to Key West? Guess what? I am sitting on the Key West Express as I write this appendix on my marathon. I'm on a 3.5-hour boat ride from Marco Island, Florida to Key West, Florida to spend another New Year's in my favorite little vacation spot in the USA. The next few days will be spent renewing my commitment to myself and my new life.

APPENDIX B - FAT CHICK

Yes, you. You're the one who is feigning not to see me when we cross paths on the running track. The one not even wearing sports gear, breathing heavy. You're slow, you breathe hard, and your efforts at moving forward make you cringe.

You cling shyly to...the furthest lane, sometimes making larger loops on the gravel ring by the track just so you're not on it, so you're not "in the way". You sweat so much that your hair is all wet. You rarely stay for more than 20 minutes at a time, and you look exhausted when you leave to go back home. You never talk to anyone. I've got something I'd like to say to you.

You are awesome!

If you'd look me in the eye only for an instant, you would notice the reverence and respect I have for you. The journey you've started is tremendous; it leads to a better health, to renewed confidence and to a brand-new kind of freedom. The gifts you'll receive from running will far exceed the gigantic effort it takes you to show up here, to face your fears and to bravely set yourself in motion in front of others.

You have already begun your transformation. You no longer accept this physical state of numbness and passivity. You have taken a difficult decision, but one that holds so much promise. Every hard breath you take is actually a tad easier than the one before, and every step is ever so slightly lighter. Each push forward leaves the former person you were in your wake, creating room for an improved version, one that is stronger, healthier and forward-looking, one who knows that anything is possible.

You're a hero to me. And, if you'd take off the blaring headphones and put your head up for more than a second or two, you would notice that the other runners you cross, the ones who probably make you feel so inadequate, are staring in awe at your determination. They, of all people, know best where you are coming from. They heard the resolutions of so many others, who vowed to pick up running and improve their health, "starting next week." Yet, it is YOU who runs alongside us, who digs from deep inside to find the strength to come here, and to come back again.

You are a runner, and no one can take that away from you. You are relentlessly moving forward. You are stronger than even you think, and you are about to be amazed by what you can do. One day, very soon, maybe tomorrow, you'll step outside and marvel at your capabilities. You will not believe your own body; you will realize that you can do this. And a new horizon will open up for you. You are a true inspiration.

I bow to you.

APPENDIX C – PROPER RUNNING FORM – BASICS (JOGGING/ RUNNING, CHI, HEAD, SHOULDERS, ARMS, FINGERS/ FISTS, TOES, CADENCE, HILLS)

This section was included as an afterthought because, while I don't care what type of cardio exercise you are doing to accomplish your healthy lifestyle, I know that running has become a big one for me. I want to impart the little knowledge that I have on the subject if (as I said from the beginning) it helps one person overcome their obesity, then it was worth it. Proper form when running is from the perspective of a fattie who didn't know what the hell jogging versus running was three years ago. Since then I've been schooled in so many areas of running, I can't quite believe it myself. I will only cover the basics I listed above because this is all most fatties will need. If you progress to the next level of running you will do the same as I did, join groups, forums, magazines (Runner's World – free plug), and enter many races.

What's jogging versus running? This is a "general rule" or "rule of thumb" so don't slay me if it's mathematically not textbook accurate. From a fattie perspective it's as accurate as it needs to be. When you're on a treadmill and you have it set to 4.4 mph or less, you are walking. I know! That's a damn fast walk – so you say. But if the stinky old, 70 – 80-year-old people at the mall can do it swinging their arms from side to side like they're actually running (but not) then your fat ass can do it too. Once you hit 4.5 mph, you're actually jogging. This will be as major of an accomplishment for you as it was for me.

Congrats. AWESOME job! Welcome to the jogging club. Keep it up and keep jogging. You will get more confident and you will get faster through speed work on a weekly (1x per week) basis. You will progress by 0.2 mph per level until you're actually doing 5.9 mph with the next level in your sites. That's right, at 6.0 mph you're actually running. If you've done the math already you'll see that 6.0 mph is actually a 10-minute per mile pace. And 4.5 mph is 75 percent of that. Once you hit 6.0 mph you're actually running. Holy shit! You rock! Good for you. You can now successfully complete a 5K in exactly 31 minutes if you can maintain that pace that long. Don't worry if you can't – you will and then you'll want "sub 30 minutes" which is technically 9:41 minutes per mile or 6.2 mph. Doesn't seem like much, does it? It is if you've never run 6.2 mph before but once you hit it and do a "sub 30," you'll weep like a baby. Most do anyway. Please send me an email when you hit your first "sub 30" as I want to share the joy with you. I'll be so proud of you. You've done amazing. Keep it up. Don't stop now!

Chi is the concept of a "controlled fall." You are leaning forward as you are running (from here forward the concept of jogging/running will be blurred but applies to both). If you're fast walking these same lessons are important, but they will become more important as you get faster. You will! It takes time. Give it time, you'll get there. There is enough of a forward "lean" (about five degrees) as you're running to show that if your next foot wasn't in front of you to take the next step/brace yourself, you'd fall flat on your face. The idea of Chi running (VERY basic - many books written on the subject) is that you need to lean into your running to use gravity as an aid in your running. You're basically continuously falling forward. The only reason you don't face plant is because your next step happens to be there before you fall. Simple, right? It is. It's just not talked about as it's assumed. If you run at a perfect 90 degrees (straight up and down) you're losing potential energy (due to wind and gravity) that you can use.

The concept of Chi is also important in running hills. I almost forgot to include this one because since I've moved to the Florida the only "hills" we have are bridges over bodies of water. They count, but barely. Basic (very basic) physics; what goes up must come down. Hills have an up slope and a down slope. Varying distances and degrees of slope, but let's KISS. There are two ways to go up a hill and two ways to come down a hill. The method you choose and the combination you choose depends on EVERYTHING from the day, the distance, the point in time the hill comes in your run, how you're feeling, etc… Going up a hill you can either slow down or attack it. There is technically a third option of maintenance, but that's pretty self-explanatory. In both approaches you should be observing maximum Chi. If you normally lean forward while running then you want even a few more degrees. If you don't normally lean forward (did you not read the last paragraph) then lean forward at least five degrees (or more). If you are going to take the hill slowly (recommended until you are accomplished at taking the hill), you should do a few simple things besides your lean. Shorten your stride even more than normal. We'll talk about cadence in a few minutes. Slow down your pace slightly (about 10 – 15 seconds) per mile or two – four steps per minute. You should do these basics (lean, shorten, slow) until you are just about to reach the crest of the hill. At that point, resume your normal lean, stride, and pace until the down slope comes. If you want to attack the hill you are going to do two-thirds of what I just said. That is, you're going to lean and shorten, but instead of slowing your pace by 10 – 15 seconds you're going to speed up your pace by 10 – 15 seconds. Why would I expend this much energy Dale? It seems counterintuitive. As I said earlier, it depends on where in the run/race the hill comes. If it's early in your run, then you should capitalize on your energy. You won't miss it later. If it's a race, you will come in ahead of your competition if you're able to attack the hills more than they are.

Let's talk about down slope. They are similar principals to ascending a hill. You can either, "recover" or "fall down" the down slope. From a form perspective you will either lean into the hill (falling) or lean back slightly (recover position). I now issue caution. If you choose to lean back slightly to recover, then you MUST make sure you read my paragraph on cadence, because leaning back will make people tend to run on their heels. This is not my intention. Just because you are leaning back does not mean your cadence/foot strike should change (see below). If you (do the opposite of running up the hill) lean back slightly, keep your stride normal, and slow your pace you will be "recovering" going down the hill, and banking some of the energy you expended going up the hill. You're overall pace won't change much because, thanks to gravity, you'll be maintaining your pace with less overall energy expenditure. If, however, you want to "speed down" or "fall down" the hill you will make up ground (similar to attacking the upslope). Your lean will once again be forward, the stride will be normal and the cadence will increase slightly (five – 10 seconds per mile). You will be flying down the hill expending the same amount of energy you would be expending on a flat road but you'll be banking time.

Cadence is the concept referred to above, but it's the **fundamental thing I advise ALL new runners** to follow no matter their level of experience. This secret is seriously worth the entire price you paid for this book. And it's located in the damn Appendix. What's up with that? It is, in my honest opinion, the SECRET to running and becoming a runner, if you're only a jogger today. It's simple and you can practice it anywhere. It's easiest to do it on a treadmill, which is how I'll explain it; but you can do it outside, just a little more challenging. You ready... ***Here's the secret: 180 steps per minute***. I don't care if you're running 6.0 mph or 10 mph. The ideal amount of times your two feet should hit the ground in one minute is 180 times. That's fairly basic, right? So 180 steps per minute (OK, now it gets a little deeper) is 90 steps per side (right versus left) in one minute. OK, that's only 180 divided by two. I got that. Easy! So, let's get on a treadmill. All treadmills have a clock to tell you how long you've been on it. As you're running on the treadmill, notice 30 seconds go by and then notice 60 seconds go by. Now that you know the secret you'll know that, ideally, your feet should be hitting the belt 180 times (or 90 per side) every minute. Let's check. OK, one more math calculation. Half of 90 is 45. Half of one minute is 30 seconds. I say this because as experience shows running and counting is easier to do over 30 seconds than a minute.

What this translates to, quite simply is that as the clock on your treadmill hits 00 at the top of a minute, you should start counting how many times your right (or left – I don't give a shit) foot hits the belt during the next 30 seconds. When the clock hits 30, check to see how close you are to 45 steps. If you hit 45 exactly, you rock, and should scream out that you are the (wo)man! If you are less than 45 then you need to shorten your stride by a distance that will allow you to hit 45 steps per side in 30 seconds. This shorter stride is the key to your future running and enjoyment of running. It corrects more things than I can write about (or care to) in this book. Lean, foot strike, energy displacement, shock to the major joints, utilization of muscle instead of bones, etc… Just trust me, if you can hit 45 steps per side in 30 seconds than you are running 180 steps per minute total. Doubt it? Count for the whole minute on one side (right or left) and see if you're hitting 90. If so, then you're doing great. Keep it up! What if you're turning over more than 180 steps per minute? I would say you have either REALLY short legs or you are Usain Bolt who turns over his feet over 200 – 210 steps every minute. The simple physics is to look at your hip girdle, and see how much energy and power you're generating from your hips to propel yourself forward. If you are insane Usain, then you're an Olympic-caliber athlete and you shouldn't be reading my book except to laugh at it, which is OK as long as you paid for it. ☺

The remaining attributes are simple (head, shoulders, arms, fingers/fists, toes) and can be summed up quickly. When running, keep your head straight and in line with your spine. Always look forward and keep your head up. When you look down at the road in front of you, you are slightly closing off your windpipe and not getting as much air into your lungs as is possible. Of course, you should look where you're going and not step in any potholes or on any rocks that will twist your ankle. Especially, if like me, you run in the early morning hours when it's dark out. You will even see me looking towards the heavens at the end of the race. While I may be praying not to collapse, more likely I'm trying to maximize the amount of oxygen I get into my lungs to fuel my heart and to pump this O_2 out to the muscles. I do this to continue to propel me forward at blinding speeds (OK, maybe not that fast but you get the point). Shoulders should be kept level just like the head. Keep them loose. Don't tense them as this will strain you and cause you to lose focus (especially on longer runs). Arms are a simple analogy. Have you ever walked across a rope bridge where it was very unsteady and you had to keep your hands on the ropes and basically pull yourself across the bridge? If not, go find a rope bridge or better yet find a YouTube video of it so you know what I'm talking about. This is what your arms should be doing. They should be going back and forth, "parallel" to the body. Your arms should NEVER cross your body at any time. Even the most experienced runner accidentally slips into this, but we all try to remember this is bad and not to do it. Again, not worth the anatomy lessen but suffice to say that when your arms are crossing your body you are putting unnecessary pressure on your interthoracic muscles (the ones around your lungs) and making them work harder then they need to in order to expand and contract (again sucking in as much oxygen as possible).

Fingers/fists – again, here's a simple anatomy. If you make a fist, it tightens up your arm muscles that tighten up your shoulder muscles that cause pain; the result is that you end up crossing them across your chest to relieve the pain. You will notice seasoned runners occasionally shaking their arms out by their sides to loosen them and their shoulders up. This is because they forgot to keep everything loose and are now having to self-adjust. It's not a bad thing to self-adjust if you screw up, but you should remember to check your form while you're running every few minutes. You will eventually remember all the things I spoke about in this paragraph and do them instinctively. Toes/feet are the same. As long as you bought proper-fitting shoes as I recommended earlier, then what you want to remember is that your toes should not be curled up in your sneakers and should always be pointing forward. Your feet should always be landing on the mid foot or ball of your foot, NEVER on the heel. This is another secret only revealed in the Appendix of this book. NEVER, EVER, allow your heel to be the first part of your foot to hit the ground when you're running. If you do, four times your body weight is being sent up from your feet to your ankles to your knee to your hips to your back. You will eventually injure yourself and not enjoy running and become fat again. Transfer your stride to your mid or ball of your foot and the "foot pounds" will be transferred to your muscles instead of your bones; and you will continue to enjoy running for many years to come.

APPENDIX D – GROUPS, RACES, COUCH TO 5K®

If you're a fattie like I was, then chances are you were embarrassed to work out or exercise in front of others; so you tended to be an introvert when it came to your exercise regimen. This means when you're doing your cardio (I'll lean towards jogging/running for the purposes of this discussion, but it can be whatever cardio you choose) you tend to do it by yourself, engrossed in your MP3 player of choice or the TV in front of the cardio machine. I am here to tell you, this is not the right path to your final destination. With that said, I will qualify the advice I'm about to give you in a few minutes. If you are jogging/running on a treadmill at the gym and following my earlier advice to ignore the others in the gym, then you've overcome your fear of going to the gym. That's great. So, when I tell you the next step in your rehabilitation is to "hit the streets" with your running/cardio, you may be as apprehensive as you were when I told you to get on the treadmill (the "mill") in the first place. It's too cold. There are cars. It's dangerous. As with so much else in this book I say to you, bullshit! Stop being such a pussy (I don't care if you're a man or woman – same phrase applies)! It's not too cold – dress in layers (I was born in Buffalo, NY and learned to run in North, NJ) – I know what cold means. Cars? Seriously, you run against traffic (or bike with traffic) so you can see them coming and they can see you (if you're biking you're going with the flow of traffic because you're a vehicle). Go to the store (local sporting goods store) and buy a couple blinking red lights to put on your shorts/shirt for late evening or early morning runs. It's dangerous? It's only dangerous if you think the treadmill is the only way to get you to your final destination. You need to physically hit the streets because just like I mentioned earlier – your body will figure out what you're doing and you have to keep it guessing.

OK, jumping ahead. Now that you've started to do some of your runs outside you will gradually see the benefits of it. TRUST ME! It took me a long time to believe this to. It's being offered to you as rock solid advice (part of the value of you reading this book). You need to NOT have a belt running under your feet so your body knows what it's like to "push off" with every step instead of a "mill" forcing you to step forward. It's better to feel wind resistance so you know what it's like when you are ready for your first race. Once you're outside you can start to incorporate hills into your workouts. Now that I've got you outside running on a regular basis, it's time for another big leap that I was also hesitant to do. Have you ever heard of RRCA? It stands for Road Runner Clubs of America. Chances are there's a Road Runner club near you, if you live near a city anywhere in the USA. If you are not sure you can always go on the Internet to www.rrca.org and click "Find a Running Club." This is the first way. A second method is to find your local sporting goods store (even better if you have an actual running store near you – if so go there first) and ask them if there's a local running club. Sometimes local clubs choose not to be associated with RRCA because there are dues involved. Totally understandable, but this shouldn't limit your ability to hook up with a good group. Why do I need to hook up with a group Dale? Because, as you start to run longer and longer, you will find the motivation and inspiration of a running group is indispensable. You will not want to come out of your comfortable introverted state. HOWEVER, once you start running with others you will find yourself sharing your story about your journey from FAT to PHAT and they will be in awe.

This will do two major things. It will inspire you to keep going and not stop because positive reinforcement is always a good thing. Secondly, it will put you "out there." Remember what I said earlier in the book about signing up for a race like a 5K. I told you to make it public and advertise the fact that you're doing it. It makes you less likely to back down. Running with a group and receiving positive reinforcement does the same thing. Once you feel like you're a part of a group, you won't want to let the group down by returning to your FAT ways. AND, you will develop a set of friends that you may not have previously had. Listen to this part, especially if you followed or understood any of the various 12-step things I've mentioned in this book. Developing a "support group" for your new, positive, healthy choices is 100 percent more likely to reinforce the behavior than not having a supportive group of similarly minded people around you. Honestly, while you may love your friends and family, chances are they are part of the problem, not part of the solution. A new "kindred spirit" group may be just the trigger you need to shift your behavior to a new paradigm. Lastly, along these same lines I mentioned a copy righted group above, "Couch to 5K®." This is a book and a movement that takes former "couch potatoes" and helps them get to their first 5K. I've coached a similar program at my local running store (maybe your local store has one or you could suggest they start one). It's the same concept as a running group except that the group is often comprised of similar fatties who want to change their lives for the better. This includes you. See if you can find one of these programs close to you as well. You will sometimes see them advertised as C25K (or go to www.c25k.com). You can download the app and do it yourself or find other like-minded slobs who've made the right choice.

APPENDIX E – SINCERE APOLOGY… KIND OF…

This appendix was a last-minute addition. It'll be brief but poignant. Here goes. Realize this is almost as difficult for me to write as the previous sections/chapters. I have beaten the shit (literally and figuratively) out of your fat ass over the last several hundred pages. But guess what, if you've made it this far it's time to see the other side of Dale. I mentioned I'm a Gemini, right? If you could see my face as I'm writing this section you would know I'm reflecting on calling you a series of horrible things, all of which you deserve. You were lazy, fat, and unmotivated, a classic obese American. If you've reached this far in the book I want to believe (I have to believe) you have or are set on changing your ways. For that, I'm emotionally grateful and humbled by your awesome display of commitment to yourself. You are a champion. You have or are about to kick ass and I will be there with you in spirit. If you can take all this advice (or at least some of it to heart), you will have had as positive impact on me as I hope I've had on you. You rock! Thank you for listening to my rants and my positive punishment and negative reinforcement. You have made it and you deserve the new life you've embarked upon. Nothing and no one will stop you. If you get stuck, remember it's a slow road and you must continue to make positive, healthy choices. There will always be people there to support you making the right decision. Depending on the outcome of sales of this book, I hope to even create a feedback forum where I can keep in touch with the people who've read and understood and embodied my words. Your commitment to yourself brings a tear to my eye. Thank you for your time and patience. Thank you for listening to my cathartic rhetoric. The first three people who read this book and lose greater than or equal to the 85 pounds (like I did) will receive a small token of my personal appreciation. Trust me, it'll be small, that is, not expensive or worth anything in a pawn shop; but it will be genuine and meaningful. You must PROVE IT and it has to have been AFTER reading the book. If that's you, get in touch with me and apply for the prize. I wish you peace and calm in your life. Namaste!